To Celeste,

My friend, colleague and collaborater.
Thanks for all your support.

Fondly yours,
Martha

Fine Needle Aspiration Biopsy of the Pancreas

Fine Needle Aspiration Biopsy of the Pancreas

Barbara A. Centeno, M.D.
Assistant Professor of Pathology, Harvard Medical School,
Boston; Assistant Pathologist, Massachusetts General Hospital,
Boston

Martha Bishop Pitman, M.D.
Assistant Professor of Pathology, Harvard Medical School,
Boston; Assistant Pathologist and Director, Fine Needle Aspira-
tion Biopsy Service, Massachusetts General Hospital, Boston

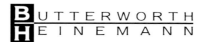

Boston • Oxford • Johannesburg • Melbourne • New Delhi • Singapore

Recognizing the importance of preserving what has been written, Butterworth–Heinemann prints its books on acid-free paper whenever possible.

 Butterworth–Heinemann supports the efforts of American Forests and the Global ReLeaf program in its campaign for the betterment of trees, forests, and our environment.

Library of Congress Cataloging-in-Publication Data
Centeno, Barbara A.
    Fine needle aspiration biopsy of pancreas / Barbara A. Centeno,
Martha Bishop Pitman.
       p.   cm.
    Includes bibliographical references and index.
    ISBN 0-7506-9725-3
    1. Pancreas--Needle biopsy. I. Pitman, Martha Bishop.
II. Title.
    [DNLM: 1. Biopsy, Needle--methods. 2. Pancreatic Neoplasms-
-diagnosis. 3. Pancreas--cytology. 4. Pancreas--pathology. WI
810 C397f 1998]
  RC857.5.C38 1998
  616.3'707582--dc21
  DNLM/DLC
  for Library of Congress   97-52016
                                             CIP

British Library Cataloguing-in-Publication Data
A catalogue record for this book is available from the British Library.

To my mother, Maria, and father, René

BAC

To Peter, Sarah, and Katherine

MBP

Contents

Contributing Authors

David P. Beech, B.A., C.T. (ASCP)
Technical Director, Cytopathology Laboratory, Massachusetts General Hospital, Boston

William R. Brugge, M.D.
Assistant Professor of Medicine, Harvard Medical School and Massachusetts General Hospital, Boston; Associate Physician, Gastrointestinal Unit, Massachusetts General Hospital, Boston

Barbara A Centeno, M.D.
Assistant Professor of Pathology, Harvard Medical School, Boston; Assistant Pathologist, Massachusetts General Hospital, Boston

Peter F. Hahn, M.D., Ph.D.
Associate Professor of Radiology, Harvard Medical School, Boston; Assistant Radiologist, Massachusetts General Hospital, Boston

Peter R. Mueller, M.D.
Associate Professor of Radiology, Harvard Medical School, Boston; Division Head, Abdominal Imaging and Interventional Radiology, Department of Radiology, Massachusetts General Hospital, Boston

Martha Bishop Pitman, M.D.
Assistant Professor of Pathology, Harvard Medical School, Boston; Assistant Pathologist and Director, Fine Needle Aspiration Biopsy Service, Massachusetts General Hospital, Boston

Daniel M. Quirk, M.D., M.P.H.
Research Fellow in Medicine, Harvard Medical School, Boston; Clinical and Research Fellow in Medicine, Massachusetts General Hospital, Boston

J. Mark Ryan, M.B., F.R.C.R., F.F.R.R.C.S.I.
Clinical Fellow, Division of Abdominal Imaging and Interventional Radiology, Department of Radiology, Massachusetts General Hospital and Harvard Medical School, Boston

Preface

This book is intended for clinicians, pathologists, fellows, residents, and cytotechnologists who are presently involved with or interested in learning about fine needle aspiration biopsy (FNAB) of the pancreas. The book provides an overview of many of the diseases that may be encountered using pancreatic FNAB, as well as pertinent clinical, radiologic, gross, and histopathologic features. The focus of the book, however, is on the cytopathologic criteria and differential diagnoses of various benign and malignant entities, illustrated by numerous color images. An emphasis is also placed on pitfalls and problem areas of diagnosis, including ways to avoid them when applicable. A unique feature of this book is the inclusion of recent advances in the diagnosis of pancreatic diseases, including criteria for the diagnosis of pancreatic adenocarcinoma, pancreatic cyst fluid analysis, and endoscopic ultrasound-guided (EUS) FNAB, which is gaining popularity at our institution.

At the Massachusetts General Hospital, rapid interpretations of deep-seated lesions are made using a modified Hematoxylin and Eosin stain; the remaining alcohol-fixed slides are stained by the standard Papanicolaou method. Air-dried slides are rarely made for Romanowsky stains, as we rely greatly on the evaluation of nuclear detail in the interpretation of the material. All three staining methods are illustrated in this monograph but with an emphasis on the alcohol-based stains. The figure legends report the objective power used to take the photograph. Any additional magnification provided by an optivar is listed adjacent to the objective power.

BAC
MBP

Acknowledgments

The editors are grateful to Drs. Peter H. Hahn, J. Mark Ryan, Peter R. Mueller, William R. Brugge, Daniel M. Quirk, and David P. Beech for contributing Chapters 1–3 and 9.

We greatly appreciate the contribution of photographs and slides from Drs. Carolyn Compton, William J. Frable, Celeste Powers, Henry Frierson, Antonio Perez-Atayde, Jan F. Silverman, James Cappellari, and Edmund S. Cibas. Dr. Kent Lewandrowski's editorial comments on pancreatic cyst fluid analysis are also greatly appreciated.

Special thanks go to Joanne Schiavo for her superb secretarial assistance and to Steve Conley and Michelle Forrestall for their photographic assistance.

Finally, we extend our thanks to our families and the pathology department for their support.

Fine Needle Aspiration Biopsy of the Pancreas

Image-Guided Pancreatic Biopsy: Development, Indications, and Complications

J. Mark Ryan, Peter F. Hahn, and Peter R. Mueller

DEVELOPMENT

Lebert was the first to publish the technique of percutaneous tumor puncture in 1851. Over the subsequent eight decades, however, little interest in the idea developed [1]. Lebert's work also included measurement of the intracellular nuclei and nucleoli of malignant cells, and he later reported an observed increase in the nuclear-to-cytoplasmic ratio in many types of tumor cells. As with his idea of tumor puncture, it was many years before the importance of his observations was recognized.

Martin and Ellis were the first to describe the actual clinical use of cytologic analysis of tissue obtained by percutaneous needle aspiration [2]. For many years, the technique remained a tool useful only for the assessment of palpable tumors and was ignored completely by North American workers. The development of modern imaging methods soon changed this trend.

Swedish workers were enthusiastic about fine needle aspiration biopsy (FNAB) of palpable tumors from the earliest reports, and they played a primary role in the subsequent development and refinement of the technique. In 1966, Dahlgren and Nordenstrom were the first to report the use of FNAB of lung tumors under fluoroscopic guidance [3]. Fluoroscopy alone was not suitable for image-guided pancreatic biopsy, and 6 years later, Oscarson et al. described the use of selective angiography as a guide for percutaneous FNAB of the pancreas [4]. This work was given further credence by the findings of Tylen et al. [5], who obtained a positive diagnosis in 22 of 29 patients with pancreatic carcinoma who were biopsied under selective angiographic guidance. Smith et al. were the first group in the United States to use ultrasound (US) as the guidance mode of choice for FNAB of intra-abdominal tumors [6]. Currently, US and computed tomography (CT) have replaced selective angiography as the primary guidance modalities for FNAB of the pancreas, but the basic technique remains essentially unchanged.

INDICATIONS

In the majority of cases, percutaneous FNAB of the pancreas is used to confirm or exclude the presence of malignancy, most commonly adenocarcinoma, suspected on clinical grounds or from prior imaging studies. Less common pancreatic neoplasms (e.g., neuroendocrine tumors, cystadenomas) and non-neoplastic lesions (e.g., pseudocysts, abscesses, cystadenomas, acute or chronic pancreatitis) can also be diagnosed using this technique.

Pancreatic cysts are a common and heterogeneous group of lesions. Neither clinical nor imaging criteria can reliably diagnose these lesions preoperatively or distinguish between benign and malignant cysts. Some studies on pancreatic cysts have investigated the pancreatic cyst fluid obtained by FNAB; by cytologic examination; and by measurement of viscosity, isoenzymes, enzyme levels, and tumor markers. Early results suggest that cyst fluid analysis can assist in differentiating malignant cystic tumors and potentially malignant mucinous cystic neoplasms from benign lesions, such as pseudocysts and microcystic adenomas [7, 8]. Pancreatic cyst fluid analysis is discussed in detail in Chapter 6.

Another important use of FNAB is as an investigative tool in the management of allograft rejection of solid organs. Allen et al. reported a diagnostic accuracy rate of 70% for the use of percutaneous FNAB in the investigation of rejection of bladder-drained pancreatic transplant [9]. An 8% false-positive rate was reported in this study. Diagnosis of early rejection was made from the detection of a patchy mononuclear cell infiltration, local destruction or loss of acinar cells with or without polymorphonuclear leukocytes, and associated capillary or venular endotheliitis. Cytologic features of late rejection included extensive mononuclear cell infiltrate, endotheliitis involving arteries and arterioles, and interstitial exudative changes, all of which were associated with widespread necrosis of the parenchyma, including necrosis of ducts, islets, and nerves.

Improvements in lesion detection, the development of a vast array of needle biopsy techniques, and changes in cytologic analysis have led to increased use of radiologically guided percutaneous biopsy. The diagnostic accuracy of percutaneous biopsy is now 80–95% [10].

FNAB of the pancreas is a minimally invasive procedure that in experienced hands facilitates the rapid assessment of a suspicious pancreatic lesion with a low complication rate. In many cases, FNAB obviates the need for a major surgical procedure, such as a diagnostic laparotomy, as shown by the study of Evander and colleagues, in which 13 of 88 patients avoided this procedure due to negative FNAB results [11].

Examination of the specimen by a cytologist at the time of biopsy enables the radiologist to know the adequacy of the specimen obtained, thus reducing the number of inadequate samples and preventing unnecessary needle passes from being performed after a satisfactory specimen has been obtained and therefore decreasing the procedural risk [12]. From initial assessment of the specimen, the cytologist can also decide what further special preparations and stains are likely to be most useful in making a definitive diagnosis.

A tissue diagnosis using FNAB prevents unnecessary surgery in the case of benign lesions and allows preoperative radiotherapy to be given in the case of malignant operable pancreatic lesions. A definitive pathologic diagnosis, combined with diagnostic imaging studies, facilitates procedure planning by the surgical team and allows a full explanation to be given to a patient before operation.

CONTRAINDICATIONS

The contraindications for FNAB of the pancreas are similar to the contraindications for FNAB of any intra-abdominal organ and are relative rather than absolute. The most important contraindication is the presence of an uncorrectable bleeding disorder, such as thrombocytopenia, a coagulopathy, or diffuse intravascular coagulation. When the urgent need for a tissue diagnosis outweighs the risk of an adverse outcome, a biopsy may proceed in the presence of an incompletely corrected bleeding diathesis.

A second relative contraindication for FNAB of the pancreas is the absence of a suitable safe access route, meaning that a bowel or a vascular structure is positioned between the proposed puncture site and the lesion to be biopsied. This problem is usually surmountable because anterior, posterior, and lateral approach routes can be used, and transgression of bowel, liver, or vascular structures with small-gauge needles is associated with very low morbidity.

PREBIOPSY PATIENT ASSESSMENT

The purpose of prebiopsy assessment is to detect any abnormality that may predispose the patient to a complication during or after the biopsy and to reduce this risk to an acceptable level (Table 1-1). Hemostatic assessment before biopsy usually follows local protocol. One study suggested that the most useful method for identifying patients with a bleeding diathesis is to obtain a full clinical history [13]. In the absence of an abnormality in the clinical history, obtaining a prothrombin time and a platelet count is sufficient for routine testing. At our institution, if the clinical history is unremarkable, we do not perform any prebiopsy coagulation assessment. For patients with known or suspected bleeding abnormalities or who have been taking anticoagulation medications, a full laboratory workup is performed.

Before performing an image-guided biopsy, the radiologist must review the patient's previous imaging studies and choose a suitable access route. Consideration should be given to the patient's mobility and ability to remain in position for the duration of the procedure.

An essential consideration important for biopsy of the pancreas is patient cooperation, which can usually be obtained readily from adult patients who have normal mental status. Careful preprocedural explanation and some intravenous sedation and analgesia can enhance a patient's ability to cooperate. For uncooperative patients and children, general anesthesia may be required.

If the patient requires general anesthesia, it must be ensured that both anesthesiologist and nursing facilities will be available at the time scheduled for the procedure.

Taking time to fully explain the procedure to the patient and answer the patient's questions is time well spent, as it reduces the patient's natural anxiety and increases his or her willingness to cooperate. Consent is obtained from the patient at this time. The patient should be advised to fast before the procedure because iodinated contrast medium may be required. Arrangements should also be made with a family member or friend to ensure that patients who have a biopsy performed on an outpatient basis can get home under supervision after the procedure. The majority of pancreatic biopsies done at our institution are performed on an outpatient basis.

TABLE 1-1. Prebiopsy Considerations

Patient's ability to cooperate
Patient size (computed tomography vs. ultrasound)
Size and location of the lesion and intervening structures
Specific lesion to be biopsied
Tumor vascularity
Needle length and caliber
Patient positioning
Available procedure room time and likely procedure length
Informed consent given
Previous cytologic or histologic studies
Presence of contraindications
Previous medical treatment
Past medical history

COMPLICATIONS

Complications may occur during or after any interventional procedure. FNAB of the pancreas may be associated with hemorrhage, pancreatitis, peritonitis, sepsis, and needle track seeding, although these complications are uncommon and rarely fatal.

The most common complications arising from FNAB of the pancreas are hemorrhage and pancreatitis. Bleeding is usually minor and self-limiting. Pancreatitis is usually transient, although there have been reports of severe pancreatitis of several months' duration [14]. The incidence of pancreatitis is approximately 3% [15]. The cause of pancreatitis occurring after FNAB has not been determined [16]; however, violation of an obstructed pancreatic duct is the most likely cause. Acute hemorrhagic pancreatitis has been reported as a fatal outcome of FNAB [17]. A case of fatal septic shock due to *Streptococcus* infection developing 8 days after aspiration of a pseudocyst has been reported, leading the authors to advise the use of prophylactic antibiotics in patients undergoing pancreatic cyst aspiration [18].

Minor complications include pain, minor hematoma formation, and vasovagal reactions. These are easily dealt with as long as the patient is carefully monitored and the process is followed to its resolution. In our institution, where most biopsies are performed on an outpatient basis, the patient is observed for 2–4 hours after the procedure. The patient should be released into the care of a responsible person who should accompany the patient home and be immediately available to the patient should any problem arise. On discharge, the patient is provided with an information sheet and an emergency contact number.

It has been shown in clinical practice that the passage of a small-gauge needle (20-gauge and smaller) through a loop of bowel is not usually associated with any complications. This may not be true, however, of larger-gauge needles, which may be associated with a higher complication rate. Therefore, caution must be exercised when using large-gauge needles. Biopsy of cystic lesions through intervening large bowel should also be avoided due to the risk of infecting the fluid contents of the cyst, thereby producing an abscess.

Tumor spread after FNAB has been reported rarely [19]. One study suggested that peritoneal washings of patients with pancreatic carcinoma who had undergone FNAB of the pancreas were more likely to be positive for malignant cells than those of patients who had not undergone a biopsy procedure [20]. This led the authors to suggest that FNAB should be avoided in patients with potentially curable disease, but the results of this study remain controversial.

Spread of malignancy along the needle tract has been reported as a rare complication of FNAB in clinical practice [21]. Some authors, however, speculate that seeding occurs more often than reported cases suggest, but these cases remain undetected clinically [16]. Studies have also demonstrated that pancreatic biopsy does not adversely influence survival rates in patients with inoperable pancreatic carcinoma [22].

At our institution, pancreatic biopsy remains a commonly performed procedure for patients with a suspicious pancreatic lesion. Patients who are scheduled for potentially curative surgery on the basis of imaging findings, dual-phase helical CT, and angiography receive 1,000 Gy of local radiotherapy before FNAB. Prebiopsy radiotherapy of 1,000 Gy does not affect cytologic interpretation of the biopsy specimen.

FNAB of the pancreas in patients with pancreatic transplant has been shown to be a safe procedure, and there are no reports of transplant failure as a result of biopsy [9, 23].

REFERENCES

1. Lebert H. Traité pratique des maladies cancereuses. Bailliere (Paris), 1851.

2. Martin HE, Ellis EB. Aspiration biopsy. Surg Gynaecol Obstet 1934;59:578.

3. Dahlgren S, Nordenstrom B. Transthoracic needle biopsy. N Engl J Med 1967;276:1081.

4. Oscarson J, Stormby N, Sundgren R. Selective angiography in fine-needle aspiration cytodiagnosis of gastric and pancreatic tumors. Acta Radiol Diagnosis 1972;12:737.

5. Tylen U, Arnesjo B, Lindberg L, et al. Percutaneous biopsy of carcinoma of the pancreas guided by angiography. Surg Gynaecol Obstet 1976;142:737.

6. Smith EH, Bartrum RJ, Chang YC. Percutaneous biopsy of the pancreas under ultrasonic guidance. N Engl J Med 1975;292:825.

7. Lewandrowski KB, Southern JF, Pins MR, et al. Cyst fluid analysis in the differential diagnosis of pancreatic cysts: a comparison of pseudocysts, serous cystadenomas, mucinous cystic neoplasms, and mucinous cystadenocarcinoma. Ann Surg 1993;217:41.

8. Lewandrowski KB, Lee J, Southern JF, et al. Cyst fluid analysis in the differential diagnosis of pancreatic cysts: a new approach to the preoperative assessment of pancreatic cyst lesions. AJR Am J Roentgenol 1995;164:815.

9. Allen RD, Wilson TG, Grierson JM, et al. Percutaneous biopsy of bladder-drained pancreas transplants. Transplantation 1991;5:1213.

10. Brandt KR, Charboneau JW, Stephens DH, et al. CT- and US-guided biopsy of the pancreas. Radiology 1993;187:99.

11. Evander A, Ihse I, Lunderquist A, et al. Percutaneous cytodiagnosis of carcinoma of the pancreas and bile duct. Ann Surg 1978;188:90.

12. Paksey N, Lilleng R, Hagmar B, et al. Diagnostic accuracy of fine needle aspiration cytology in pancreatic lesions. A review of 77 cases. Acta Cytol 1993;37:889.

13. Silverman SG, Mueller PR, Pfister RC. Hemostatic evaluation before abdominal intervention: an overview and proposal. AJR Am J Roentgenol 1990;154:233.

14. Mueller PR, Miketic LM, Simeone JF, et al. Severe acute pancreatitis after percutaneous biopsy of the pancreas. AJR Am J Roentgenol 1988;151:493.

15. Yankaskas BC, Staab EV, Craven MB, et al. Delayed complications from fine-needle biopsies of solid masses of the abdomen. Invest Radiol 1986;21:325.

16. Smith EH. Complications of percutaneous abdominal fine-needle biopsy. Radiology 1991;178:253.

17. Levin DP, Bret PM. Percutaneous FNAB of the pancreas resulting in death. Gastrointest Radiol 1991;16:67.

18. Ulich TR, Layfield LJ. Fatal septic shock after fine-needle aspiration of a pancreatic pseudocyst. Acta Cytol 1985;29:879.

19. Weiss SN, Skibber JM, Mohiuddin M, et al. Rapid intraabdominal spread of pancreatic cancer. Arch Surg 1985;120:415.

20. Warshaw AL. Implications of peritoneal cytology for staging of early pancreatic cancer. Am J Surg 1991;161:26.

21. Smith FP, MacDonald JS, Schein S, et al. Cutaneous seeding of pancreatic cancer by skinny needle aspiration biopsy. Arch Intern Med 1980;140:855.

22. Balen FG, Little A, Smith AC, et al. Biopsy of inoperable pancreatic tumors does not adversely influence patient survival time. Radiology 1994;193:753.

23. Bernardino M, Fernandez M, Neylan J, et al. Pancreatic transplants—CT-guided biopsy. Radiology 1990;177:709.

Pancreatic Fine Needle Aspiration Biopsy: Imaging, Equipment, and Technique

J. Mark Ryan, Peter F. Hahn, and Peter R. Mueller

LESION LOCALIZATION AND CHOICE OF MODALITY FOR RADIOLOGICALLY GUIDED PANCREATIC FINE NEEDLE ASPIRATION BIOPSY

Exact localization of the lesion to be biopsied is central to the successful performance of radiologically guided pancreatic biopsy. Several imaging modes are available for imaging guidance of percutaneous fine needle aspiration biopsy (FNAB). In each case, the simplest imaging system providing adequate definition of the mass and adjacent structures and allowing safe and accurate insertion of the needle into the lesion should be used. For pancreatic FNAB, ultrasound (US) and computed tomography (CT) are generally the preferred guidance techniques. Each technique provides a cost-effective option.

Personal preference and the radiologist's expertise with a modality are important factors. The availability of the modality for the duration of the procedure should be considered because difficult biopsies can use a procedure room for a prolonged time. In most cases, however, size and location of the lesion dictate which modality is employed. At Massachusetts General Hospital, the majority of FNABs of the pancreas are performed using CT guidance. This reflects the pattern of referral to our interventional radiology service, however, because most lesions are small and percutaneous access routes tend to be challenging.

Both US and CT have the advantages of direct visualization of the region to be biopsied and three-dimensional localization of the needle within the lesion (Table 2-1). Low-echogenicity areas on US and low-attenuation areas on CT may represent areas of necrosis within a tumor. Both CT and US can show features of the internal structure of a mass, and if areas of necrosis are suspected, a region of the lesion considered more likely to yield the most information can be targeted. The periphery of a lesion most often yields diagnostic information because it is the area least likely to be affected by tumor necrosis.

A study by Brandt and coworkers reported that the accuracy rate for diagnosing pancreatic carcinoma by FNAB was 86% for CT-guided biopsies and 95% for US-guided biopsies [1, 2]. These results may reflect a degree of unavoidable selection bias because larger lesions are well demonstrated by US and therefore quickly and easily biopsied under US guidance, whereas the smaller and more difficult lesions are preferentially biopsied using CT guidance. With US, scanning can be performed in multiple planes, and tumor size, depth, and texture can be readily assessed. US-guided biopsy is technically more difficult than CT-guided biopsy, and the operator must have considerable experience with real-time scanning.

Although fluoroscopy-guided biopsy in conjunction with angiography has been superseded by US and CT, the use of fluoroscopy for biopsy of the pancreas has not been abandoned entirely. Because tumors of the pancreatic head tend to present with biliary obstruction, the highest biopsy yield may be obtained at the point of biliary duct narrowing. Thus, the use of fluoroscopy to guide needle aspiration of a narrowed segment of duct in conjunction with cholangiography, or after placement of a biliary stent, remains a valuable but infrequently used technique (Figure 2-1).

ULTRASOUND-GUIDED FINE NEEDLE ASPIRATION BIOPSY

The US probes used for percutaneous biopsy are usually in the range of 3.5–7.0 MHz. When the biopsy needle is

TABLE 2-1. Comparative Advantages of Ultrasound and Computed Tomography

Ultrasound	Computed Tomography
Rapid localization	Better resolution
Portable capability	Identifies needle tip
Flexible positioning	Lack of bowel-gas artifact
No radiation	Precise anatomic detail
Identifies needle tip–tumor relationship in real time	
Inexpensive	

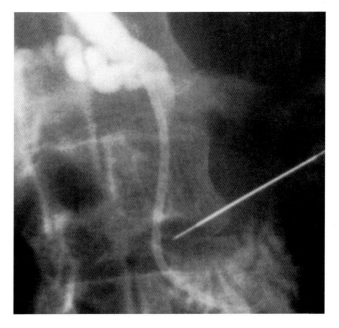

FIGURE 2-1. Fluoroscopy-guided biopsy of pancreatic head lesion. The patient has a biliary stent in situ that is used as a target during needle insertion. A cholangiogram demonstrates dilatation of the proximal common bile duct and cystic duct.

perpendicular to the incident sound waves, it reflects the sound waves at an angle equal to the incident sound waves, thereby giving maximum needle visibility. Needle conspicuity is directly related to transducer frequency; therefore, the highest-frequency transducer that allows adequate lesion visualization should be used. Reduction in transducer size from technological advancements means that the site of the lesion and the availability of a sonographic window determine the choice of transducer rather than overall transducer size, as was previously the case.

Some refinement of the US-guided technique has occurred over the last decade with the development of a dedicated linear array transducer with a slotted needle aperture and the sector scanner with the disposable sterile snap-on device for needle guidance (with or without the accompanying computer software). This "needle guide" technique is not commonly used at our institution because we prefer the more versatile freehand method using a standard transducer.

The freehand method entails preparing a sterile field around the proposed puncture site. The transducer is placed into a sterile plastic sleeve with coupling gel. The radiologist, wearing sterile gloves, gown, and eye protection, holds the biopsy needle in one hand and the US transducer in the other. The needle is held at right angles to the transducer and is advanced into the mass to be biopsied, during which time the needle-tip position is monitored in

real time. Slight to-and-fro movement of the needle helps to localize the needle tip if there is uncertainty. This technique requires greater skill than the needle guide technique but, once mastered, offers greater flexibility than the needle guide technique. Some radiologists prefer to use the needle guide method because they believe that it allows quicker and more accurate needle placement. An ongoing study in our department does not support this belief.

A disadvantage of the use of US for pancreatic biopsy is that difficulty in visualizing the pancreas can be encountered if the bowel is gas filled or the patient is obese (fat strongly attenuates the US beam, thereby diminishing lesion conspicuity). Pancreatic tail lesions can also be particularly difficult to visualize with US.

COMPUTED TOMOGRAPHY–GUIDED FINE NEEDLE ASPIRATION BIOPSY

FNAB of the pancreas using CT guidance is technically easier than US and is not limited by some of the disadvantages of US (see Table 2-1). CT-guided FNAB also offers the versatility of a posterior approach, as well as facilitates a more detailed anatomic representation of the region to be biopsied and of the intervening structures. Unlike US, the image is not degraded by the presence of bowel gas; however, CT-guided pancreatic biopsy is usually a more time-consuming procedure.

FIGURE 2-2. Computed tomography–guided biopsy of a pancreatic mass. The needle tip is seen in the mass.

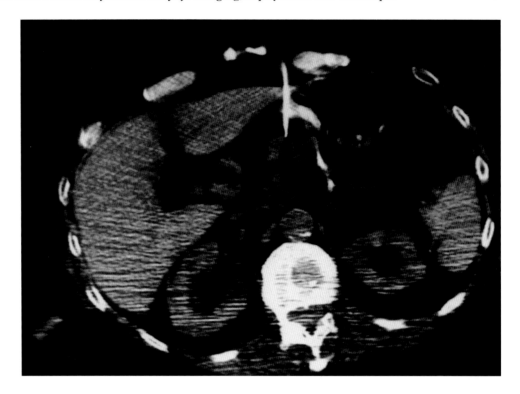

FIGURE 2-2. Computed tomography–guided biopsy of a pancreatic mass. The needle tip is seen in the mass.

After a prebiopsy imaging study has identified the lesion to be biopsied, the area of interest is re-examined with a radiopaque grid on the patient's skin. The site of entry is marked with a sterile marker, and the grid is then removed. A sterile area is prepared, and a total of 10–15 ml of 1% lidocaine is administered into the skin and subcutaneous and deep tissues. The biopsy needle is then inserted to the predetermined length ascertained from the initial scan, and the region is rescanned with the needle in position (Figure 2-2). Adjustment of the needle depth is performed, if necessary, and an additional localizing scan is obtained. If the initial biopsy needle is determined to be in a suboptimal position, a second biopsy needle is inserted into a more optimal position, with the first needle used as a reference point. This is called the *tandem technique*. A needle that is perpendicular to the x-ray beam permits better visualization of the needle tip, but angulation of the needle creates only minor difficulties in identifying the needle tip. The position of the needle tip can be confirmed by the presence of a characteristic streak artifact (Figure 2-3); however, this artifact is less prominent with newer helical scanners.

Hence, a major drawback of CT for FNAB is the lack of real-time monitoring of the needle tip, which contributes to the time-consuming nature of the procedure. Some newer-generation CT scanners do offer a capacity for real-time imaging of the needle, but they are not yet widely available. This method also contributes to a relatively high radiation dose to the radiologist, and its value remains unproven.

MAGNETIC RESONANCE–GUIDED BIOPSY

Percutaneous magnetic resonance (MR)-guided biopsy has been available for several years, and dedicated interventional MR units have been developed for this purpose. It is uncommon for MR to be required for percutaneous biopsy of intra-abdominal lesions, the main benefit for MR-guided biopsy being stereotactic biopsy of the head and neck. Specialized nonferromagnetic needles and marking grids are required for biopsy using MR localization, and these biopsy systems are now commercially available to a limited degree. The procedure is costly, and the precise value of the technique in the abdomen remains uncertain. As a result, MR-guided pancreatic biopsy is performed in some institutions on an experimental basis but is not widely used in clinical practice.

BIOPSY TECHNIQUE

After infiltration of local analgesia into the skin and superficial tissues, a small skin nick is made with a No. 11 blade. This facilitates easier insertion of the needle

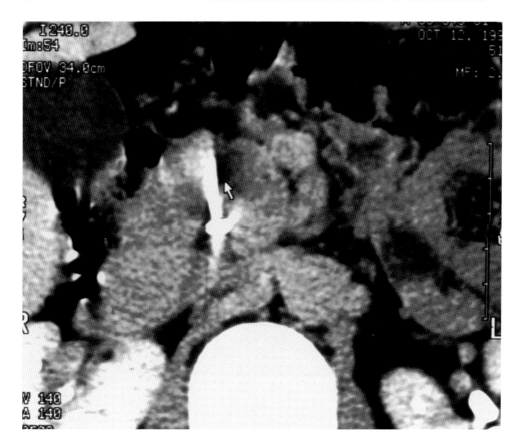

FIGURE 2-3. Computed tomography–guided biopsy of another pancreatic head lesion with biopsy needle in position. Needle tip artifact is seen. The patient has a biliary stent in situ. The arrow points to the low-density tumor.

and reduces the resistance that is encountered in the superficial tissues, which can cause deviation of the biopsy needle from its intended path. Real-time scanning with US allows small adjustments to be made to the path of the needle according to the visual information on the screen. During advancement of the needle for CT-guided biopsy, angulation of the needle must be monitored, with the tabletop as a reference point and comparison made with the initial localizing scan. Adjustments can be made to needle position if necessary, using the tandem technique described above.

Once the needle is in optimal position, as determined by imaging, the inner stylet of the needle is removed. A specimen is obtained by attaching a 12-ml syringe to the needle and applying a rotational drilling motion to the needle and syringe with one hand, while suction is applied to the plunger and depth of needle insertion is controlled with the other hand. A locking mechanism between the syringe and needle maximizes control during rotation and suction. The successful performance of this maneuver requires practice and experience. Special biopsy systems, including a vacuum syringe, have been developed to make the maneuver less complicated and to facilitate easier and more constant application of suction to the syringe.

The tissue sample lodges in the shaft of the needle, and the needle is withdrawn after releasing suction on the plunger. The sample is expelled onto a slide, and smears are prepared using the two-slide pull-apart technique. Residual particulate matter is suspended in saline for subsequent cell block preparation and analysis.

BIOPSY NEEDLES

Needle Selection

A variety of biopsy needles and needle systems of different caliber, length, and tip design are commercially available for FNAB. They are referred to as either small (20- to 22-gauge) or large (18-gauge) needles. The smaller-gauge needles are generally thought to be associated with lower risk of complications than the larger-gauge needles. This belief is supported by both clinical [3] and experimental studies [4]. Bowel and vascular structures can be punctured with smaller-gauge needles with little associated risk, but these needles may be less consistent than larger-gauge needles in obtaining adequate tissue for cytologic examination [5]. Generally, smaller-caliber needles are preferred for FNAB of the pancreas [6].

Multiple punctures are permitted with smaller-caliber needles because of a lower complication rate. These needles are preferred when the track of the needle violates the pleura, a vascular structure, or bowel. It is also advisable to use a small-caliber needle in the pres-

FIGURE 2-4. (A) Chiba needle. (B) Chiba tip design demonstrated.

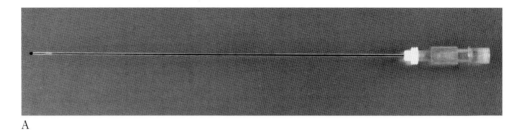

A

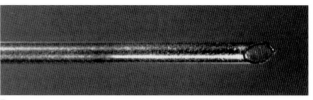

B

ence of a known bleeding diathesis. Smaller-gauge needles are usually adequate for the confirmation of tumor recurrence or metastases from documented previous malignancy. Tissue cores may be required by the cytologist, and these are more reliably obtained by larger-gauge needles. The 22-gauge needles may deflect when resistance is encountered in the superficial or deep tissues; therefore, stiffer 20-gauge needles offer greater resistance to deflection and hence greater control.

If an initial attempt with a 22- or 20-gauge needle has not provided sufficient material for cytologic analysis, an additional pass is made with an 18-gauge needle, with the position of the smaller-gauge needle used as a guide. The use of large-gauge needles improves the yield of both cytologic and histologic material. Fewer needle passes should be performed with large-gauge needles because of the slightly increased risk of hemorrhage associated with their use.

Needle Tip Design

The Chiba needle (Medi-tech/Boston Scientific, Natick, MA) was the original workhorse needle for FNAB. Most subsequent developments in needle design are modifications of the original Chiba needle. The needle tip, the angle of the bevel, and the cutting edge of the bevel have all been modified in an attempt to gain better cytology and tissue core specimens. FNAB needles are generally categorized as either aspiration or cutting needles and are available in different lengths and calibers. The choice depends on the depth of the lesion to be biopsied and the type of specimen required.

The Chiba (Figure 2-4) and Turner needles (Cook Inc., Bloomington, IN) (Figure 2-5) are both aspiration needles. The Chiba has a 25-degree bevel and is available in 20- to 23-gauge sizes. The Turner needle has a 45-degree bevel at the tip; its design is thought to facilitate the acquisition of better core specimens for histologic examination. It is commercially available in 16-, 18-, 20-, and 22-gauge sizes.

Cutting-type needles, such as the Franseen (Medi-tech/Boston Scientific) (Figure 2-6) and the Greene (Cook Inc.) (Figure 2-7), are designed to increase the probability of obtaining an adequate histologic specimen as well as cytologic material. The Franseen needle, with its cutting serrated tip, is designed to optimize aspiration of a tissue core and fragments with needle rotation.

Commercial coaxial biopsy systems, such as the Greene biopsy set (Cook Inc.) and the vanSonnenberg modified coaxial biopsy set (Cook Inc.) are now widely available and are commonly used. The rationale behind the use of these coaxial systems is that a larger needle is used for localization and stabilization of the lesion, and multiple passes with the smaller-caliber needle are made through the larger needle. This obviates the need for multiple passes of the needle through vascular or intestinal structures. The coaxial technique is ideally suited for biopsy of deep lesions and therefore applicable to FNAB of the pancreas.

CONCLUSION

FNAB of the pancreas is a commonly performed procedure that is usually done using US or CT guidance. It is

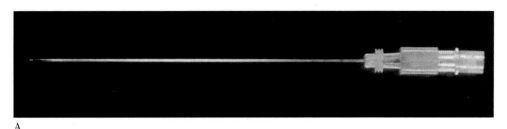

A

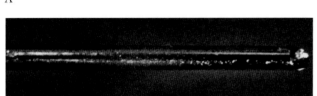

B

FIGURE 2-5. (A) Turner needle. (B) The Turner needle has a diamond-tipped stylet with a beveled needle tip.

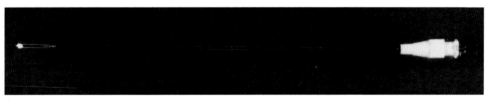

A

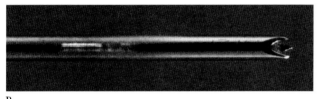

B

FIGURE 2-6. (A) Franseen cutting needle. (B) Tip design of the Franseen needle.

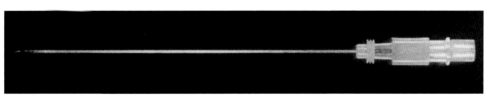

A

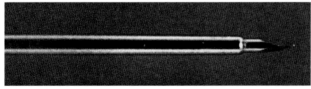

B

FIGURE 2-7. (A) Greene needle. (B) The tip is circumferentially sharpened.

associated with a low complication rate. The successful performance of FNAB requires a sound understanding of radiologic imaging and its limitations and of the technical aspects of needle selection, needle placement, and specimen procurement.

REFERENCES

1. Brandt KR, Charboneau JW, Stephens DH, et al. CT- and US-guided pancreatic biopsy. Radiology 1993;187:99.

2. Philips VM, Hersch T, Erwin BC, et al. Percutaneous biopsy of pancreatic masses. J Clin Gastroenterol 1985;7:506.

3. Welch TJ, Sheedy PF, Stephens DH et al. Percutaneous adrenal biopsy: review of a 10-year experience. Radiology 1994;193:341.

4. Gazelle GS, Haaga JR, Rowland DY. Effect of needle gauge, level of anticoagulation, and target organ on bleeding associated with aspiration biopsy. Radiology 1992;183:509.

5. Haaga J, LiPuma JP, Bryan PJ, et al. Clinical comparison of small- and large-caliber cutting needles for biopsy. Radiology 1983;146:665.

6. Wittenberg J, Mueller PR, Ferrucci JT, et al. Percutaneous core biopsy of abdominal tumors using 22 gauge needles—further observations. AJR Am J Roentgenol 1982;139:75.

Endoscopic Ultrasonography–Directed Fine Needle Aspiration

Daniel M. Quirk and William R. Brugge

Endoscopic ultrasonography (EUS) has undergone many refinements since its introduction in 1982. The initial radial scanning instruments allowed for detailed imaging of the esophageal and gastric walls as well as adjacent structures, such as lymph nodes, the pancreas, and the bile duct [1]. As a result of the extensive experience with this instrument, evaluations of submucosal abnormalities, cancer staging of luminal tumors, and evaluation of pancreaticobiliary disease, including pancreatic cancer staging, have become established indications [2]. The advent of the linear array echoendoscope (Pentax Precision Instruments Corp., Orangeburg, NY) has made it possible to perform needle aspiration biopsies of mural and extramural lesions [3–8].

INDICATIONS

Experience with EUS-directed fine needle aspiration (EUS-FNA) is growing rapidly, and early results have been quite promising. The potential indications for EUS-FNA include diagnosis of the primary lesion, lymph node staging, and biopsy of distant metastatic sites, such as the liver [2].

CONTRAINDICATIONS

The principal component of EUS-FNA is upper endoscopy. As such, the contraindications for the procedure are similar to those of upper endoscopy. Absolute contraindications include the patient's inability to cooperate with the examination, structural lesions that prohibit the passing of the echoendoscope into the desired location, severe shock, and respiratory distress [9]. EUS-FNA has been complicated by bleeding in a very few instances; there-fore, it may be prudent to view coagulopathy as a relative contraindication [10, 11].

ADVANTAGES

The advantages of EUS-FNA over transcutaneous FNA are becoming more apparent as further experience with this procedure is gained. Perhaps the greatest advantage of EUS-FNA is that it allows for the biopsy of small lesions that are not evident by conventional imaging studies [3]. Lesions as small as 4 mm have been accurately biopsied with EUS-FNA [4]. A second advantage is the close proximity of the echoendoscope in relation to the target tissue. Therefore, the needle path is shorter, and the needle does not need to traverse any other intra-abdominal structures, as opposed to transcutaneous biopsy, in which the needle must pass through another structure 24–40% of the time [12]. The practical implications of this are evident, but the theoretical may be just as important. There is conflicting evidence that transcutaneous pancreatic biopsy can lead to seeding of the biopsy track [13–20]. In EUS-FNA, this concern is mitigated by the fact that the needle passes through only the duodenal or gastric wall. Therefore, even if seeding was to occur, the only tissue seeded would be part of the surgical resection specimen, as opposed to other abdominal organs or cutaneous tissue. Another advantage of EUS-FNA is that it can be performed at the time of initial staging, thereby not requiring a second procedure, with its costs.

PREBIOPSY ASSESSMENT

The prebiopsy assessment is similar to that for percutaneous aspirates and includes a history, physical examina-

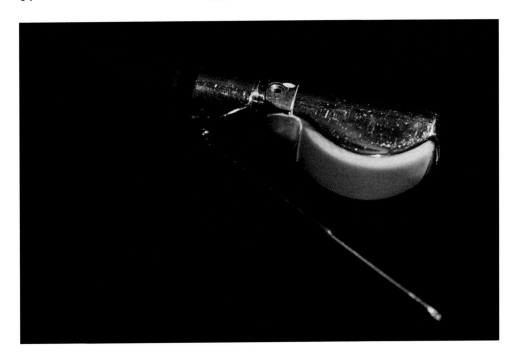

FIGURE 3-1. Tip of the Pentax FG-32UA echoendoscope (Pentax Precision Instruments Corp., Orangeburg, NY) with needle exiting from biopsy channel.

tion, and selected laboratory studies if indicated. The history and physical examination should be used to ascertain if there is evidence of medication allergy, bleeding diathesis, cervical arthritis, valvular heart disease, esophageal obstruction, or possible gastric outlet obstruction. If the history or physical examination suggest the possibility of a bleeding diathesis, a prothrombin time and platelet count should be checked before biopsy [9].

COMPLICATIONS

EUS is a relatively safe procedure. The reported complication rate is 0.05% [21]. The majority of reported complications are perforations associated with malignant luminal stenoses. Therefore, in the absence of such stenoses, one would expect the complication rate to be even lower. EUS-FNA is associated with a complication rate of 0–2% [10, 11]. This rate compares favorably to the 3.3% rate reported for percutaneous pancreatic biopsy [12]. To date, the associated complications with EUS-FNA have included fever, infection, perforation, bleeding, and pancreatitis.

EQUIPMENT

The current image guidance system consists of the Pentax FG-32UA echoendoscope (Pentax Precision Instruments Corp.) in conjunction with the Hitachi EUB-515C ultrasound console (Mitsubishi, Conshohocken, PA). The endoscope is 160 cm long, with a diameter of 10.8 mm. The optics are oriented in the 60-degree oblique forward direction with a 110-degree viewing field. The

ultrasound transducer is mounted distal to the viewing optics. The transducer measures 36 mm long and 12 mm wide. The scanning plane is in the long axis of the endoscope at an angle of 100 degrees. The scanning frequency is 5.0 or 7.5 MHz, and the penetration depth is 5–6 cm. A 2-mm biopsy channel is oriented so that the biopsy needle is advanced into the imaging plane, allowing for real-time imaging of the actual biopsy (Figure 3-1).

Many prototype needles have been developed. The GIP/Medi-Globe needle (Medi-Globe Corp., Tempe, AZ) is an excellent example. The needle is stainless steel, 180 cm in length, and 22 gauge in diameter. A beveled stylet is inserted through the entire length of the needle. The needle is enclosed in either a polytetrafluoroethylene (polytef, or Teflon) or metal sheath for safe introduction through the biopsy channel. Under ultrasound guidance, the needle can be advanced up to 5 cm beyond the sheath and into the lesion.

TECHNIQUE

The biopsy is performed after thorough endoscopic and ultrasonographic examination. Once the lesion is localized, the biopsy path is investigated to ensure that there are no vascular structures. When this is confirmed, the catheter containing the needle with stylet is introduced into the biopsy channel. The needle is advanced beyond the polytef catheter into the ultrasound field of view. The needle is then advanced through the lumen into the lesion under ultrasound guidance (Figure 3-2). Once in the lesion, the stylet is removed (Figure 3-3). A 10- to

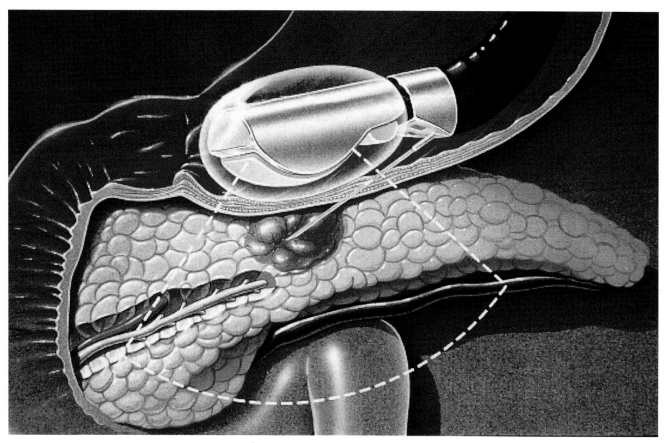

FIGURE 3-2. The Pentax FG-32UA transducer in the gastric antrum. The needle is shown exiting the biopsy channel and traversing the gastric wall into the pancreatic lesion. (Reproduced with the permission of the Pentax Precision Instruments Corp., Orangeburg, NY.)

FIGURE 3-3. Endoscopic ultrasound image of a hypoeochic pancreatic mass (*arrows*) with a biopsy needle (*N*) entering the lesion.

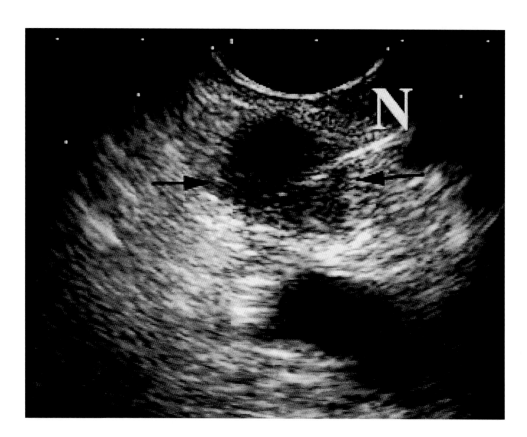

20-ml syringe is attached to the end of the needle via high-pressure tubing. Suction is then applied to the syringe, and the needle is moved to and fro inside the lesion. The vacuum is then released, the needle retracted into the catheter, and the catheter and needle removed from the biopsy channel. The aspirated material is then placed on slides for cytologic analysis. The entire procedure is repeated until adequate material has been obtained [4].

REFERENCES

1. Caletti G, Ferrari A. Endoscopic ultrasonography. Endoscopy 1996;28:156.

2. Lightdale CJ. Indications, contraindications, and complications of endoscopic ultrasonography. Gastrointest Endosc 1996;43:S15.

3. Wiersema MJ, Kochman ML, Cramer HM, et al. Endosonography-guided real-time fine-needle aspiration biopsy. Gastrointest Endosc 1994;40:700.

4. Vilmann P, Hancke S, Henriksen FW, Jacobsen GK. Endoscopic ultrasonography-guided fine-needle aspiration biopsy of lesions in the upper gastrointestinal tract. Gastrointest Endosc 1995;41:230.

5. Vilmann P, Jacobsen GK, Henriksen FW, Hancke S. Endoscopic ultrasonography with guided fine needle aspiration biopsy in pancreatic disease. Gastrointest Endosc 1992;38:172.

6. Vilmann P, Hancke S, Henriksen FW, Jacobsen GK. Endosonographically-guided fine needle aspiration biopsy of malignant lesions in the upper gastrointestinal tract. Endoscopy 1993;25:523.

7. Giovannini M, Seitz JF, Monges G, et al. Fine-needle aspiration cytology guided by endoscopic ultrasonography: results in 141 patients. Endoscopy 1995;27:171.

8. Chang KJ, Katz KD, Durbin TE, et al. Endoscopic ultrasound-guided fine-needle aspiration. Gastrointest Endosc 1994;40:694.

9. Tytgat GNJ. Upper Gastrointestinal Endoscopy. In T Yamada, DH Alpers, C Owyang, et al. (eds), Textbook of Gastroenterology. Philadelphia: Lippincott, 1995;2544.

10. Gress F, Ikenberry S, Hawes R, et al. Endoscopic ultrasound (EUS) guided fine needle aspiration (FNA) biopsy utilizing linear array and radial scanning endosonography: results of diagnostic accuracy and complications [abstract]. Gastrointest Endosc 1996;43:421.

11. Chang KJ, Wiersema M, Giovannini M, et al. Multi-center collaborative study on endoscopic ultrasound (EUS) guided fine needle aspiration (FNA) of the pancreas [abstract]. Gastrointest Endosc 1996;43:417.

12. Brandt KB, Charboneau JW, Stephens DH, et al. CT- and US-guided biopsy of the pancreas. Radiology 1993;187:99.

13. Ferrucci JT, Wittenberg J, Margolies MN, Carey RW. Malignant seeding of the tract after thin-needle aspiration biopsy. Radiology 1979;130:345.

14. Balen FG, Little A, Smith AC, et al. Biopsy of inoperable pancreatic tumors does not adversely influence patient survival time. Radiology 1994;193:753.

15. Warshaw AL. Implications of peritoneal cytology for staging early pancreatic cancer. Am J Surg 1991;161:26.

16. Schadt ME, Kline TS, Neal HS, et al. Intraoperative pancreatic fine needle aspiration biopsy results in 166 patients. Am Surg 1991;57:73.

17. Weiss SM, Skibber JM, Mohiuddin M, Rosato FE. Rapid intra-abdominal spread of pancreatic cancer. Arch Surg 1985;120:415.

18. Smith EH. Complications of percutaneous abdominal fine-needle biopsy. Radiology 1991;178:253.

19. Ryd W, Hagmar B, Ericksson O. Local tumor cell seeding by fine-needle aspiration biopsy: a semiquantitative study. APMIS 1983;91:17.

20. Ericksson O, Hagmar B, Ryd W. Effects of fine-needle aspiration and other biopsy procedures on tumor dissemination in mice. Cancer 1984;54:73.

21. Rosch T, Dittler HJ, Fockens P, et al. Major complications of endoscopic ultrasonography: results of a survey of 42,105 cases [abstract]. Gastrointest Endosc 1993;39:341.

CHAPTER

4

Normal Pancreas

Martha Bishop Pitman

EMBRYOLOGY

The pancreas begins as two buds arising from the duodenal endoderm; their fusion at 7 weeks forms the pancreas. The smaller ventral bud, originating from the developing hepatic duct, forms the inferior part of the pancreatic head and uncinate process. The larger dorsal bud, developing from the opposite side of the foregut, forms the remainder [1, 2]. Anastomosis of the distal part of the dorsal pancreatic duct with the ventral pancreatic duct produces the duct of Wirsung, the major excretory duct. The proximal dorsal pancreatic duct is obliterated or persists as the duct of Santorini, the accessory pancreatic duct (Figure 4-1) [3]. The islets of Langerhans develop from the pancreatic parenchyma at 12 weeks' gestation [2].

ANATOMY

The normal adult pancreas averages 15 cm in length and 100 g in weight [3]. It is partially retroperitoneal, with the pancreatic head nestled in the curve of the duodenum and the tail abutting the hilum of the spleen. Surrounding structures include the splenic artery superiorly, duodenum medially, diaphragm anteriorly, and inferior vena cava posteriorly [4]. The primary blood supply is from the superior mesenteric artery and branches of the celiac trunk. Venous drainage occurs via the hepatic portal system. Lymphatics accompany the blood vessels.

HISTOLOGY

The pancreas comprises both exocrine (80%) and endocrine (20%) components [3].

Exocrine Component

The exocrine component consists of ductal and acinar elements, the latter forming the majority of the exocrine pancreas. Coalesced acini form lobules separated by thin strands of connective tissue. Individual acini are composed of pyramidal to columnar acinar epithelial cells with a basal nucleus arranged around a tiny, often invisible lumen. The apical region contains numerous periodic acid–Schiff (PAS)-positive secretory (zymogen) granules, which lend coarse granularity to the cytoplasm (Figure 4-2).

The duct system, which receives the proteolytic enzymes released from the zymogen granules, begins with the centroacinar cell. Centroacinar cells connect the acini to the intercalated ducts and stand out on histology sections because of their pale, clearly defined cytoplasm and oblong nuclei when cut longitudinally (see Figures 4-2 and 4-3). The intercalated duct is lined by flattened to low cuboidal cells (see Figure 4-3). As the ducts become larger, the lining cells become increasingly taller and more columnar and eventually mucin secreting, forming the intralobular (Figure 4-4), interlobular (Figure 4-5), and main excretory ducts (Figure 4-6) [5].

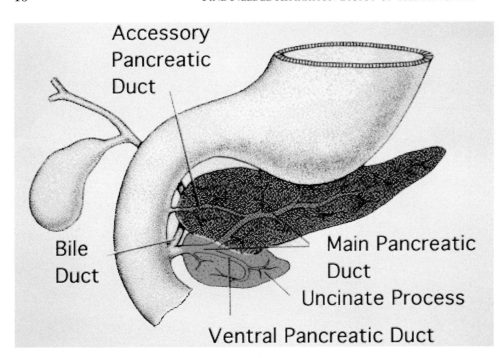

FIGURE 4-1. Embryologic development of the pancreas. The ventral pancreatic bud (*blue*) fuses with the dorsal pancreatic bud (*red*) at approximately 7 weeks. The anastomosing ducts form the major excretory duct, the duct of Wirsung. (Modified with permission from TW Sadler. Langman's Medical Embryology [6th ed]. Baltimore: Williams & Wilkins, 1990.)

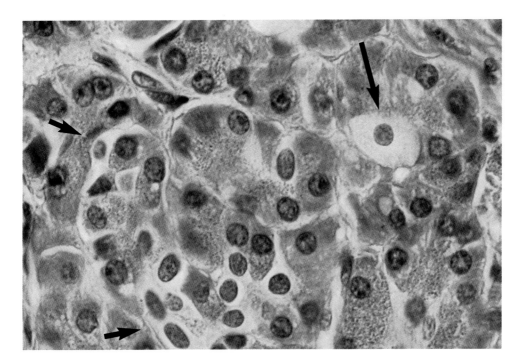

FIGURE 4-2. The exocrine pancreas. The acinar elements of the exocrine pancreas consist of polygonal cells with abundant granular cytoplasm and basal nuclei. Centroacinar cells (*arrows*) are defined by their pale cytoplasm and connect the acini to the intercalated ducts (Hematoxylin and Eosin, 100×).

FIGURE 4-3. The exocrine pancreas. Centroacinar cells have oblong nuclei when cut longitudinally (*arrowheads*) and lead to the intercalated ducts (*arrow*), which are lined by flattened to low cuboidal cells. The surrounding acinar epithelium is distinguished by its abundant, coarsely granular, eosinophilic cytoplasm (Hematoxylin and Eosin, 100×).

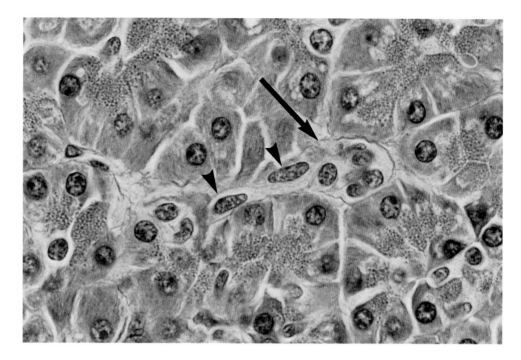

FIGURE 4-4. The exocrine pancreas. Intercalated ducts lead to the larger intralobular ducts, which are lined by slightly taller, more columnar epithelium (Hematoxylin and Eosin, 100×).

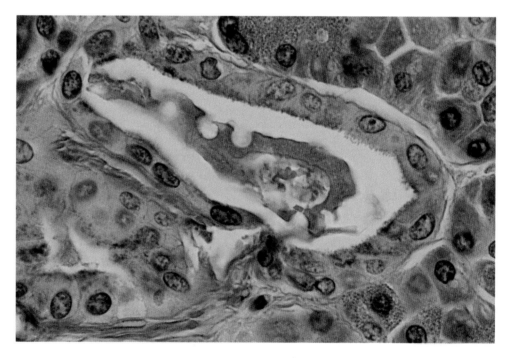

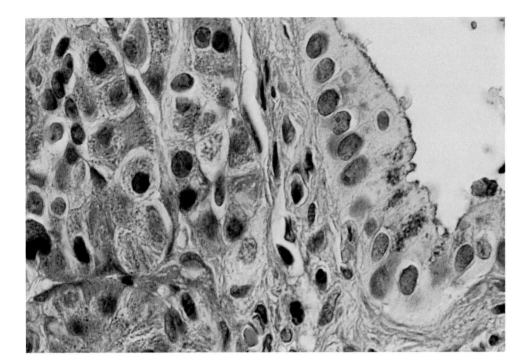

FIGURE 4-5. The exocrine pancreas. The intralobular ducts lead to the interlobular ducts, which are lined by even taller columnar epithelium (Hematoxylin and Eosin, 100×).

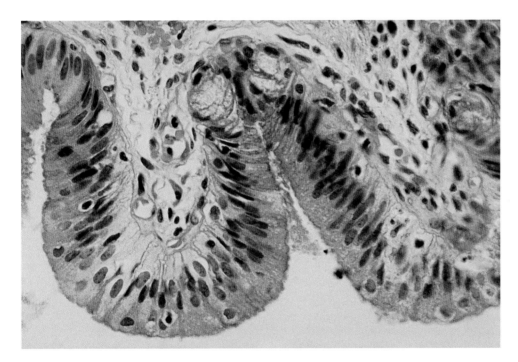

FIGURE 4-6. The exocrine pancreas. The main excretory duct is fed by interlobular ducts and is lined by mucinous columnar epithelium (Hematoxylin and Eosin, 100×).

Endocrine Component

Islets of Langerhans constitute the endocrine portion of the pancreas, representing a relatively large part of the newborn pancreas but only 1–2% of the adult pancreas [6]. Each islet is composed of a compact, rounded nest of uniform polygonal cells intimately associated with numerous capillaries (Figure 4-7) [7].

Islets arising from the ventral pancreatic bud in the uncinate process and posterior pancreatic head are slightly irregular in outline and are rich in pancreatic polypeptide [8]. The other islets are dominated by insulin-secreting cells, which are concentrated in the central regions of the islet. Glucagon-secreting cells are most numerous at the periphery, whereas somatostatin-secreting cells are randomly distributed [7].

FIGURE 4-7. The endocrine pancreas. Islets of Langerhans are composed of a compact rounded nest of uniform polygonal cells intimately associated with numerous capillaries (Hematoxylin and Eosin, 20×).

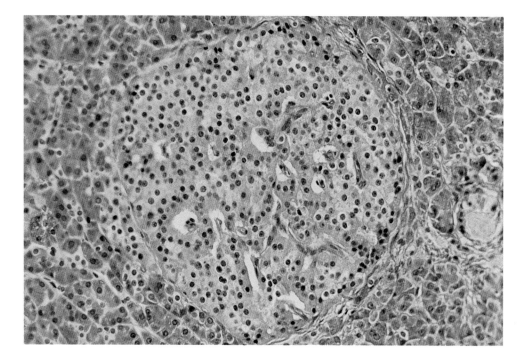

FIGURE 4-8. Cells that secrete various hormones and proteins constitute the islets and are distinguished by very subtle morphologic differences that are virtually impossible to detect on routine histologic sections (Hematoxylin and Eosin, 100×).

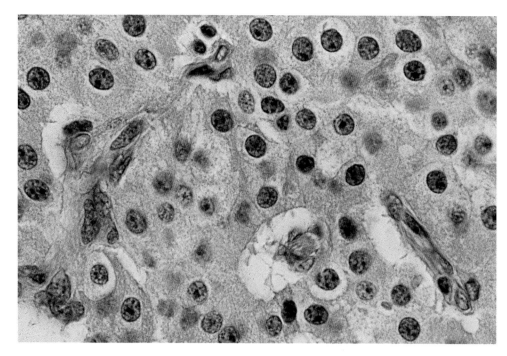

The morphologic differences in these cells are subtle and virtually impossible to detect on routine histologic sections (Figure 4-8).

CYTOLOGY

Acinar Epithelium

Acinar cells dominate cytology specimens obtained by fine needle aspiration biopsy (FNAB). Acinar cells are arranged predominantly in tightly cohesive, small, grapelike clusters and tubular groups that have a small lumen, but they may also be present singly (Figure 4-9). The pyramidal-shaped cells have ample cytoplasm that is usually dense and granular, staining blue-green with the standard Papanicolaou stain (Figure 4-10) and eosinophilic with Hematoxylin and Eosin (Figure 4-11). Air-dried May-Grünwald–Giemsa–stained preparations enhance the abundance and granularity of the cytoplasm (Figure 4-12). The nuclear detail of the

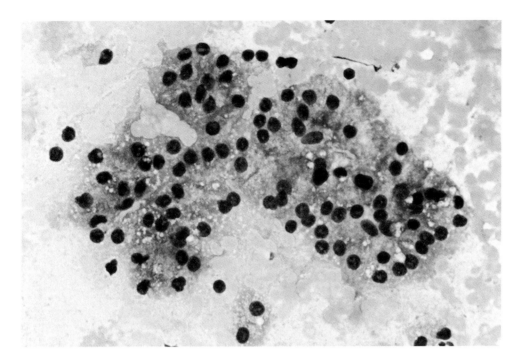

FIGURE 4-9. Fine needle aspiration smears are dominated by acinar cells, which are arranged in tightly cohesive, grapelike clusters and occasionally as single cells (May-Grünwald–Giemsa, 63×).

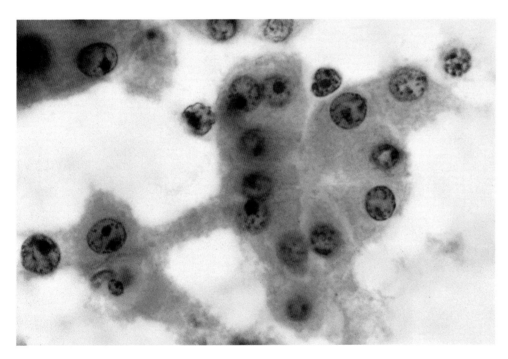

FIGURE 4-10. Acinar epithelial cells are pyramidal-shaped cells with abundant, dense, granular cytoplasm and round regular nuclei (Papanicolaou, 100×; ×1.25 optivar).

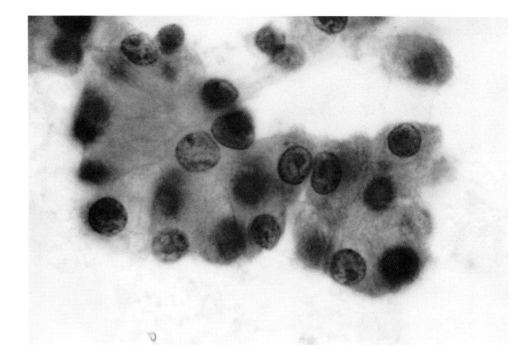

FIGURE 4-11. Acinar epithelial cells demonstrate eosinophilic cytoplasm on Hematoxylin and Eosin stain (100×; ×1.25 optivar). Note that nucleoli may be quite prominent.

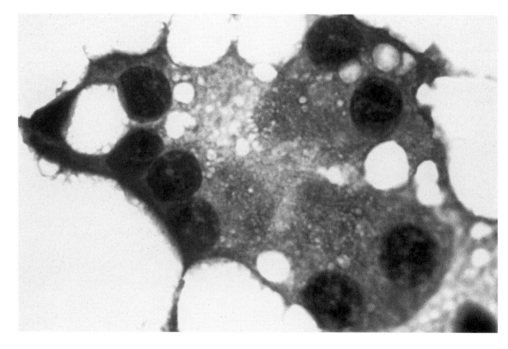

FIGURE 4-12. Air-dried smears enhance the abundance and granularity of the cytoplasm (May-Grünwald–Giemsa, 100×; ×1.25 optivar).

basally oriented nuclei is best demonstrated with alcohol fixation and either Papanicolaou or Hematoxylin and Eosin stain. The nuclei are round and regular with even, fine chromatin and nucleoli that are usually quite conspicuous (see Figures 4-10, 4-11, and 4-12).

Ductal Epithelium

The ductal epithelium present on smears is usually from the larger, interlobular ducts lined by tall, columnar epithelium. These cells may be observed in flat, mono-layered sheets with a typical glandular honeycomb pattern (Figure 4-13) or on edge, where the full columnar profile demonstrates a "picket-fence" arrangement (Figure 4-14). In both instances, the nuclei are round to oval, regular, and uniform and have a fine, evenly distributed chromatin pattern. Nucleoli are not conspicuous, as in acinar cells. Cytoplasm is best appreciated in cells seen in profile, where the tall apical cytoplasmic compartment is moderately dense and uniform, staining blue with the

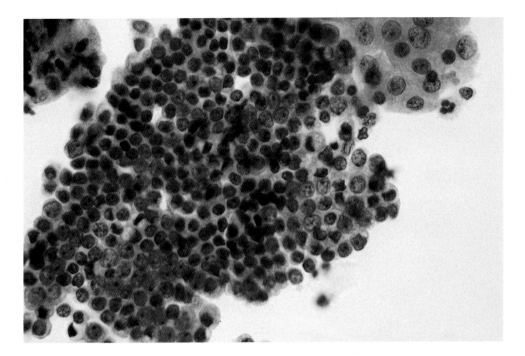

FIGURE 4-13. Ductal epithelial cells form typical glandular honeycomb sheets with nuclei in a uniform, evenly spaced distribution (Papanicolaou, 40×).

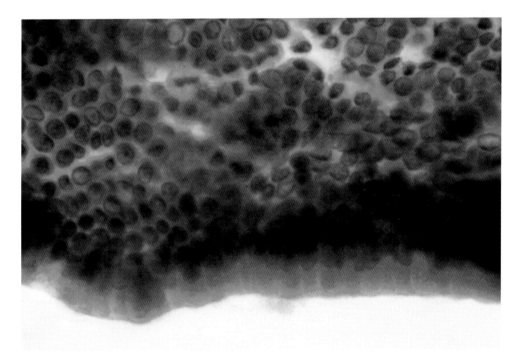

FIGURE 4-14. Ductal epithelium from the larger interlobular ducts lined by columnar epithelium may demonstrate a "picket-fence" arrangement (Papanicolaou, 63×).

Papanicolaou stain (see Figure 4-14), eosinophilic with Hematoxylin and Eosin (Figure 4-15), and purple with air-dried May-Grünwald–Giemsa stain (Figure 4-16).

Islets of Langerhans

Cells from the islets of Langerhans are rarely appreciated on FNAB smears unless, of course, the smear is of an islet cell proliferation. Aspirates of the tail of a normal pancreas at autopsy produced organoid clusters (personal observations) (Figure 4-17) and small groups (Figure 4-18) of polygonal, uniform cells with round nuclei, coarse chromatin, and indistinct cytoplasm. Some groups may closely resemble ductal cells because of focal eccentric cytoplasm (see Figure 4-18). A Grimelius stain (Figure 4-19) demonstrates the neurosecretory granules.

FIGURE 4-15. A smaller fragment of ductal epithelium on edge demonstrates columnar morphology (Hematoxylin and Eosin, 100×).

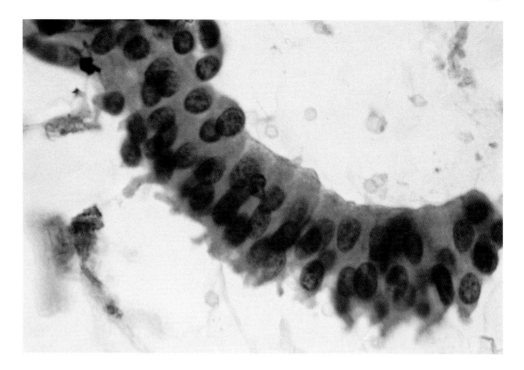

FIGURE 4-16. Small cluster of ductal epithelium shows columnar morphology (May-Grünwald–Giemsa, 100×).

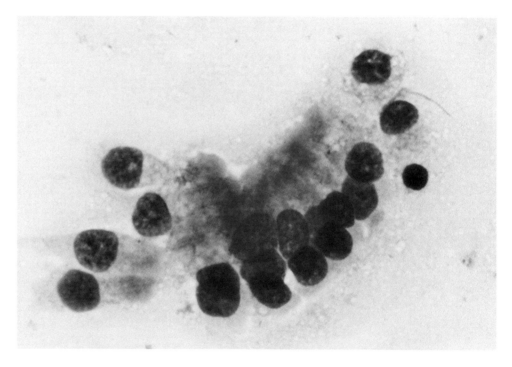

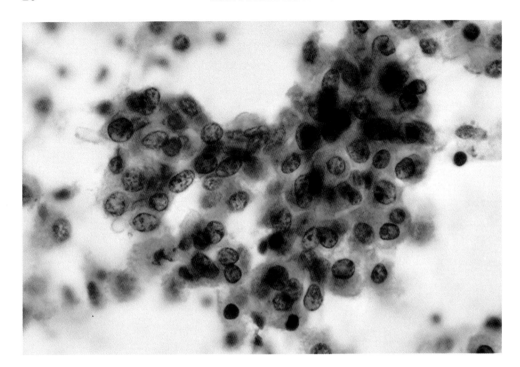

FIGURE 4-17. Organoid cluster of islet cells in an aspirate from the tail of a cadaveric pancreas (Papanicolaou, 40×).

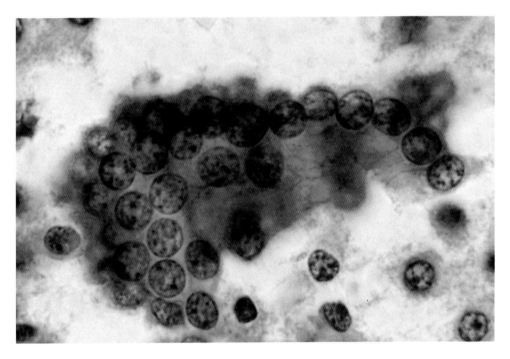

FIGURE 4-18. Islet cells are polygonal, uniform cells with round nuclei, coarse chromatin, and indistinct cytoplasm that may focally appear columnar and resemble ductal epithelium (Papanicolaou, 63×).

Contaminants

The principal contaminant in FNABs of the pancreas is mesothelium. Mesothelium occurs in large, flat, often folded monolayered sheets composed of uniform, evenly spaced cells separated by clear spaces, or "windows" (Figures 4-20 and 4-21). The small, round to oval nuclei have even chromatin and may contain visible nucleoli (see Figure 4-21). Mesothelium can easily be mistaken for ductal epithelium and may be a major pitfall in diagnosis when it is atypical in appearance (Figure 4-22) [9]. Other contaminants include hepatocytes (Figure 4-23) and gastrointestinal epithelium (Figure 4-24).

FIGURE 4-19. A Grimelius stain demonstrates the black neurosecretory granules in the cytoplasm of islet cells (Grimelius, 100×).

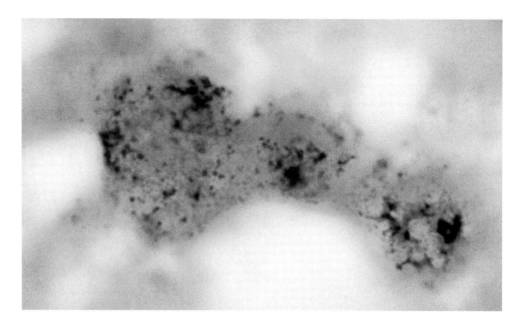

FIGURE 4-20. Reactive mesothelial cells are recognized by their flat, frequently folded, monolayered sheet arrangement with nuclei separated by "windows" (Papanicolaou, 63×).

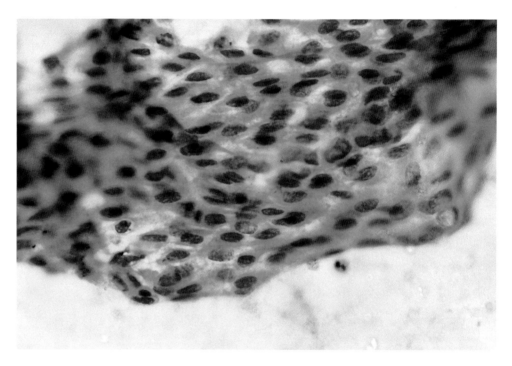

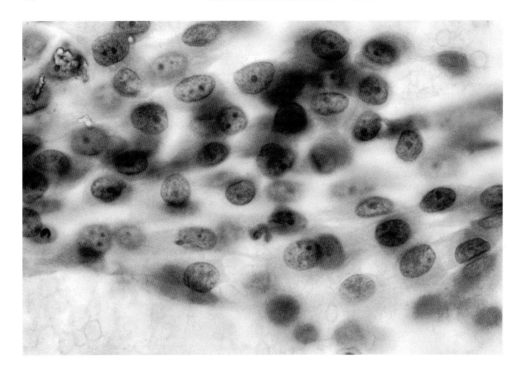

FIGURE 4-21. A higher magnification of the mesothelial cells shows small round to oval nuclei with an even chromatin pattern and visible nucleoli (Hematoxylin and Eosin, 100×).

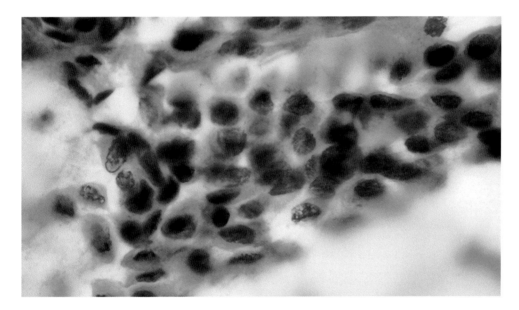

FIGURE 4-22. Markedly reactive mesothelial cells are a major pitfall of false-positive diagnoses in aspirations of the pancreas (Papanicolaou, 100×).

FIGURE 4-23. Hepatocytes are sometimes a contaminant in fine needle aspirations of the pancreas. These cells are large polygonal cells with abundant granular cytoplasm and round central nuclei that may demonstrate nucleoli (Papanicolaou, 63×).

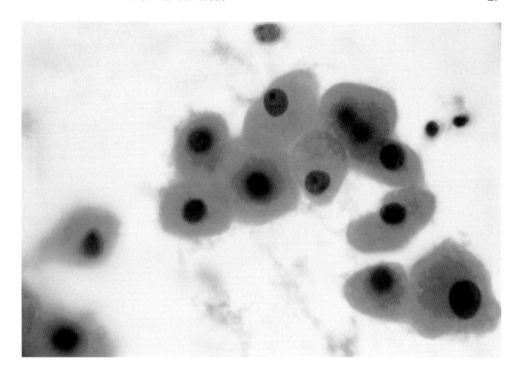

FIGURE 4-24. Gastrointestinal epithelium is also a common contaminant in fine needle aspirations of the pancreas, particularly those using endoscopic biopsy technique. It may be impossible to distinguish gastrointestinal-type epithelium from ductal epithelium (Papanicolaou, 100×).

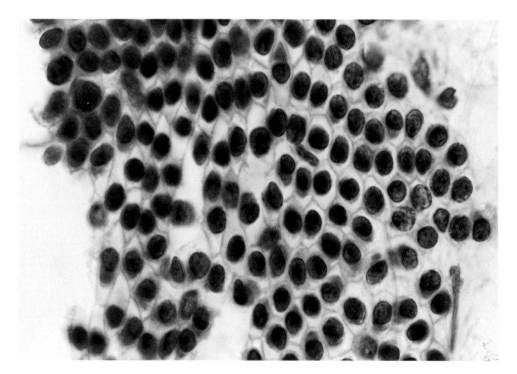

REFERENCES

1. Heitz PU, Beglinger C, Gyr K. Anatomy and Physiology of the Exocrine Pancreas. In G Kloppel, PU Heitz (eds), Pancreatic Pathology. Edinburgh: Churchill Livingstone, 1984;3.

2. Sadler TW. Langman's Medical Embryology. Baltimore: William & Wilkins, 1990;246.

3. Crawford JM, Cotran RS. The Pancreas. In RS Cotran, V Kumar, SL Robbins (eds), Robbins' Pathologic Basis of Disease (4th ed). Philadelphia: Saunders, 1989;897.

4. Williams PL, Warwick R, Dyson M, Bannister LH. The Pancreas. In P Williams (ed), Gray's Anatomy (37th ed). New York: Churchill Livingstone, 1989;1380.

5. Oertel JE, Heffess CS, Oertel YC. Pancreas. In S Sternberg (ed), Histology for Pathologists. New York: Raven, 1992;657.

6. Stefan Y, Grasso S, Perrelet A, Orci L. A quantitative immunofluorescent study of the endocrine cell populations in the developing human pancreas. Diabetes 1983;32:293.

7. Kloppel G, Lenzen S. Anatomy and Physiology of the Endocrine Pancreas. In G Kloppel, PU Heitz (eds), Pancreatic Pathology. Edinburgh: Churchill Livingstone, 1984;133.

8. Bommer G, Friedl U, Heitz PU, Kloppel G. Pancreatic PP cell distribution and hyperplasia. Immunocytochemical morphology in the normal human pancreas, in chronic pancreatitis and pancreatic carcinoma. Virchows Arch 1980;387:319.

9. Koss LG. Diagnostic Cytology and Its Histopathologic Bases (Vol 2, 4th ed). Philadelphia: Lippincott, 1992;1357.

CHAPTER 5

Pancreatitis

Martha Bishop Pitman

Pancreatitis is generally a clinically based diagnosis with no need for biopsy confirmation. Exceptions occur when pancreatitis produces a mass lesion detectable by imaging studies, which leads to investigation by fine needle aspiration biopsy (FNAB) to exclude malignancy. Inflammatory lesions, most of which center around some form of pancreatitis [1, 2], account for the majority of nonneoplastic pancreatic lesions aspirated. Pancreatitis and carcinoma commonly occur simultaneously, carcinoma being the most common cause of main pancreatic duct obstruction [3]. This association leads to difficulties in obtaining a representative sample and difficulties in the interpretation of smears.

This chapter focuses on the FNAB findings in pancreatitis and the distinction between benign, reactive ductal changes and well-differentiated ductal adenocarcinoma. Pseudocysts and other cystic inflammatory lesions are discussed in Chapter 6.

ACUTE PANCREATITIS

Most cases of acute pancreatitis are noninfectious and a result of autodigestion by the gland's own proteolytic and lipolytic enzymes [3]. Multiple factors are generally involved but broadly fall into etiologic categories of biliary disease, alcoholism and nutrition, toxic or therapeutic agents, heredity, metabolic abnormalities, and congenital or acquired structural defects [2].

Acute pancreatitis ranges from a mild, self-limited form to very severe hemorrhagic, necrotizing pancreatitis. Acute pancreatitis may also result from recurrent episodes of chronic relapsing pancreatitis.

Grossly, proteolytic destruction leads to a soft yellow parenchyma with flecks of chalky white fat necrosis (Figure 5-1). Destruction of blood vessels with subsequent hemorrhage results in hemorrhagic pancreatitis (Figure 5-2).

Although the diagnosis of uncomplicated acute pancreatitis or an acute exacerbation of chronic pancreatitis is usually a clinical diagnosis not requiring imaging studies or biopsy confirmation [4], imaging studies are often indicated when complications of hemorrhagic or necrotizing pancreatitis, pseudocyst formation, or a superimposed infection are suspected. Ultrasound (US) and computed tomography (CT) are the imaging modalities of choice, endoscopic retrograde cholangiopancreatography (ERCP) being contraindicated in acute pancreatitis [4]. The presence of diffuse pancreatic enlargement and a large fluid collection in the lesser sac is diagnostic of acute pancreatitis (Figure 5-3) [5]. Focal pancreatic enlargement or a pancreatic mass lesion may be present (Figure 5-4), however, and may be the only abnormality identified. It is these rare cases that lend themselves to evaluation by FNAB.

Aspirates are usually dominated by fat necrosis, neutrophils, and granulation tissue. These are the features that generally overshadow the earlier stages of granular coagulative necrosis caused by the initial release of the digestive enzymes of the acinar cells (Figure 5-5), the sequela of which is the potential to manifest as a focal mass lesion on imaging studies [5]. Fat necrosis of the intraparenchymal and peripancreatic adipose tissue is the result of saponification that forms calcium soaps. On aspiration smears, this is manifested by degenerating fat cells, frequently present as mere ghost cells, and variable numbers of foamy, or lipid-laden, macrophages (Figure 5-6). Neutrophilic debris is also

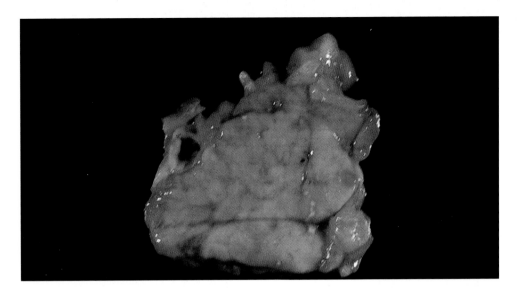

FIGURE 5-1. Acute pancreatitis. Soft yellow parenchyma contains flecks of chalky white fat necrosis.

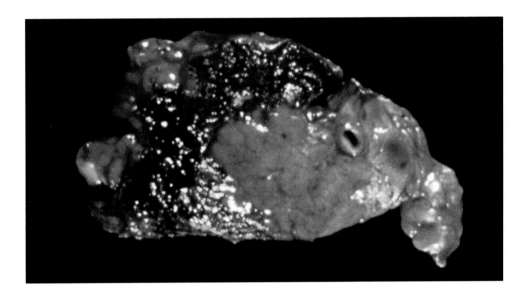

FIGURE 5-2. Hemorrhagic pancreatitis. Destruction of blood vessels leads to subsequent hemorrhage in some cases of acute pancreatitis.

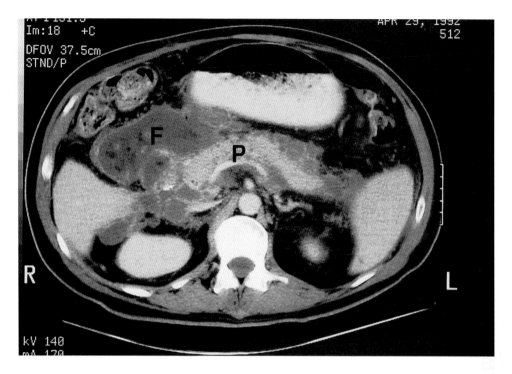

FIGURE 5-3. Computed tomographic image illustrating classic case of acute pancreatitis with diffuse pancreatic enlargement (P) and a fluid collection (F) in the lesser sac.

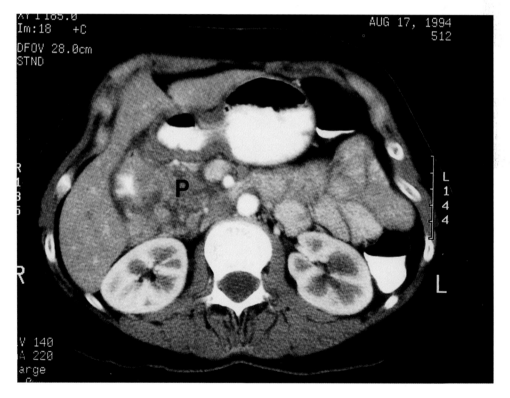

FIGURE 5-4. Focal pancreatic enlargement (P) in a case of acute pancreatitis.

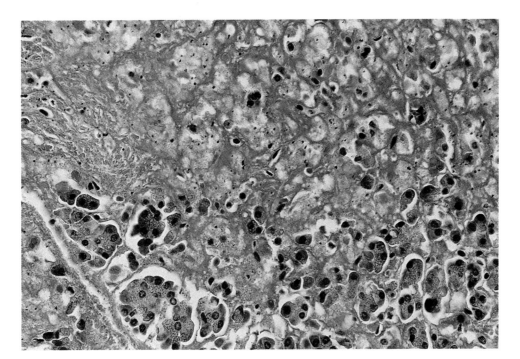

Figure 5-5. Histologic section of acute pancreatitis demonstrating marked fat necrosis and saponification (Hematoxylin and Eosin, 40×).

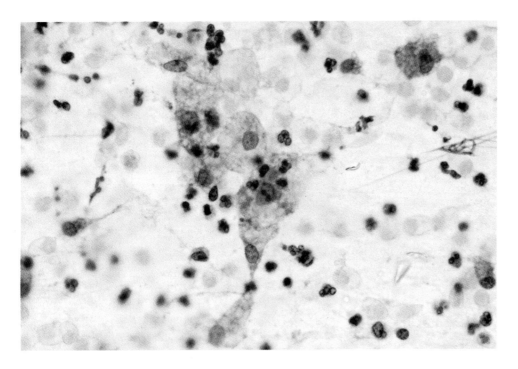

Figure 5-6. Aspiration smears of acute pancreatitis frequently show numerous foamy or lipid-laden macrophages in a background of degenerating fat cells and ghost cells (Hematoxylin and Eosin, 40×; ×1.25 optivar).

FIGURE 5-7. Coagulum of
neutrophils in acute pancreatitis (Hematoxylin and
Eosin, 40×; ×1.25 optivar).

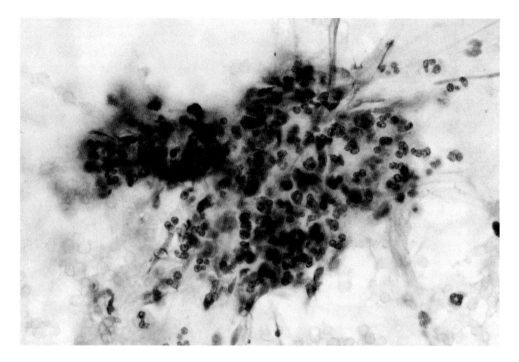

FIGURE 5-8. Aspiration
smears may show clusters
of degenerating or necrotic
ductal and acinar epithe-
lium associated with
inflammatory cells (Papanicolaou, 63×).

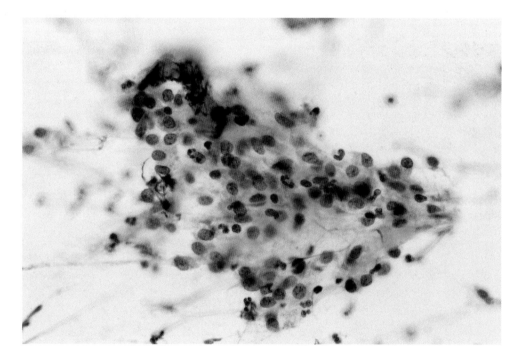

plentiful (Figure 5-7), and necrotic ductal and acinar epithelium may be present (Figure 5-8).

Granulation tissue forms during the healing and reparative process and is composed of a proliferation of capillaries, fibroblasts, and inflammatory cells. During the early active phase of healing, the granulation tissue is highly cellular and mitotically active, but during the end stages, the cellularity greatly decreases, leaving dense fibrous tissue or a scar. It is the cellular early stage that is apparent on an aspiration biopsy. Granulation tissue is manifested by a capillary network surrounded by immature fibroblasts and various inflammatory cells, including lymphocytes, plasma cells, and histiocytes (Figures 5-9 and 5-10).

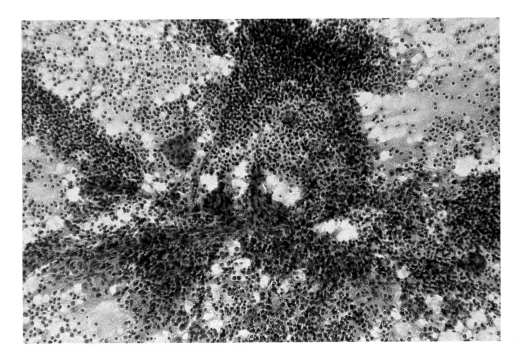

FIGURE 5-9. The healing phase of acute pancreatitis is dominated by granulation tissue, which is composed of a proliferation of small capillaries, immature fibroblasts, and various inflammatory cells, including lymphocytes, plasma cells, and histiocytes (Papanicolaou, 10×).

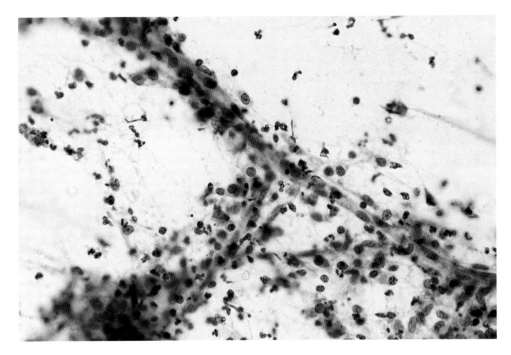

FIGURE 5-10. High-power image of granulation tissue in healing acute pancreatitis (Papanicolaou, 40×).

Cytologic Features of Acute Pancreatitis
- Early
    Degenerated (saponified) fat cells
    Foamy histiocytes
    Neutrophilic debris
    ± Necrotic ductal and acinar cells
- Healing
    Granulation tissue
        Proliferating capillaries
        Reactive, immature fibroblasts

Inflammatory cells: lymphocytes, neutrophils, and plasma cells

CHRONIC PANCREATITIS

The typical manifestations of chronic pancreatitis detectable with contrast-enhanced current-generation CT examination include pancreatic ductal dilatation, parenchymal atrophy, and pancreatic calculi [4]. The presence of calcifications

FIGURE 5-11. Computed tomographic image showing needle placed within focal pancreatic enlargement (*P*) in chronic pancreatitis. The black line (to the left of the P) is a reflection off the needle tip (white blurry line) at the edge of the mass.

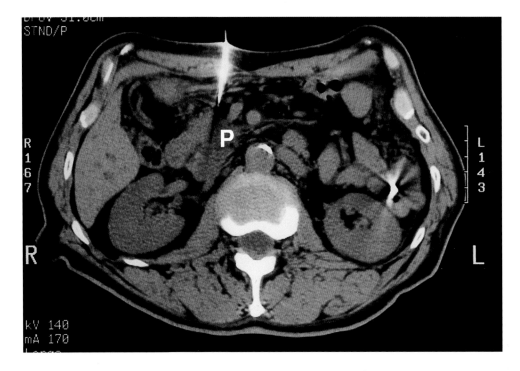

FIGURE 5-12. The cut surface of the pancreas in chronic pancreatitis shows a dense, firm parenchyma due to fibrosis.

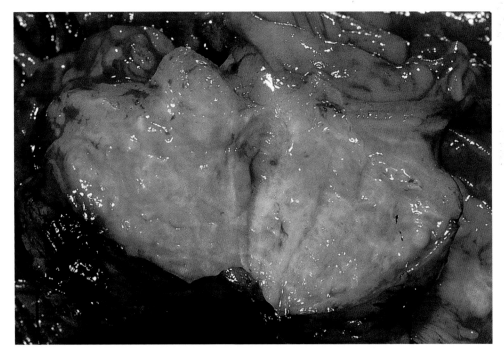

on CT helps to distinguish between benign and malignant disease. Extensive, diffusely scattered ductal calculi within the mass are virtually pathognomonic of an inflammatory enlargement [4]. Focal pancreatic enlargement has been reported in more than 30% of cases of chronic pancreatitis [4], thus raising the question of malignancy (Figure 5-11). This indeterminate mass must be evaluated with a tissue diagnosis, FNAB being widely accepted as the diagnostic procedure of choice. The FNAB may be performed percutaneously, intraoperatively, via ERCP, or using endoscopic ultrasound guidance.

Grossly, chronic pancreatitis results in a smaller gland with firm, dense parenchyma due to fibrosis and scarring (Figure 5-12). The cause of chronic pancreatitis that results in an indeterminate mass lesion is generally

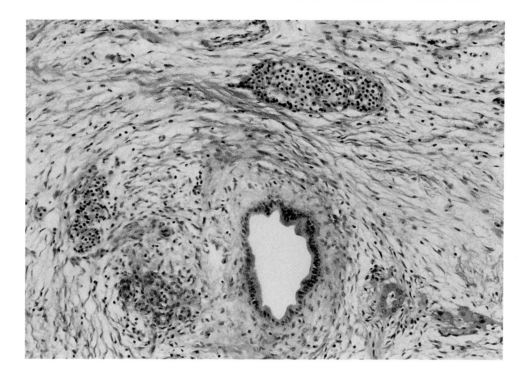

FIGURE 5-13. The histology of chronic pancreatitis varies depending on the degree of fibrosis that has destroyed the exocrine portion of the pancreas and spared the isolated islands of islet cells (Hematoxylin and Eosin, 10×; ×1.25 optivar).

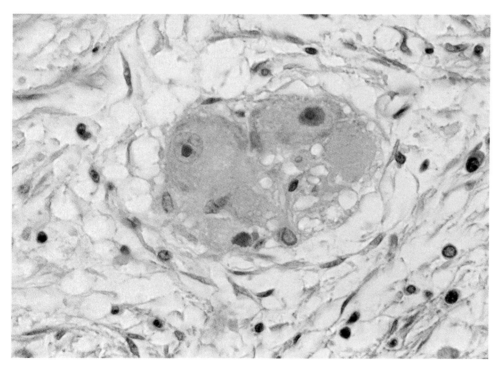

FIGURE 5-14. Histologic section of chronic pancreatitis illustrating residual atypical but reactive acinar epithelium embedded in fibrous tissue (Hematoxylin and Eosin, 40×; ×1.25 optivar).

obstruction [6]. In this form of chronic pancreatitis, the distribution of destructive lesions is irregular rather than lobular, as in the calcifying form of chronic pancreatitis commonly associated with an alcoholic etiology. The exocrine pancreas in both forms is damaged, resulting in atrophy of the acinar epithelium, interlobular fibrosis, and a chronic inflammatory cell infiltrate around lobules and ducts. The islets of Langerhans are remarkably spared (Figure 5-13) [3]. Residual acinar cells may be quite atypical, with nuclear pleomorphism and prominent nucleoli (Figure 5-14).

The overall cellularity of smears in chronic pancreatitis varies depending on the degree of fibrosis. Although generally not hypercellular, smears from

FIGURE 5-15. Chronic active pancreatitis. The smear is dominated by ductal epithelium but also contains clusters of acinar epithelium and numerous inflammatory cells (Papanicolaou, 10×).

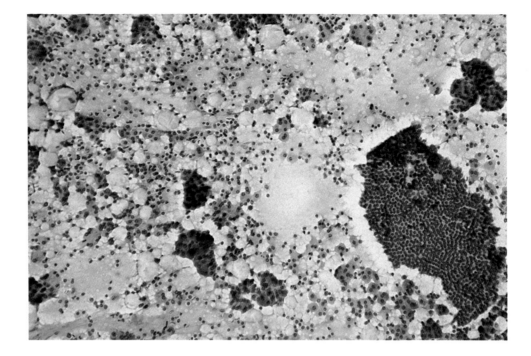

FIGURE 5-16. Chronic pancreatitis. A sheet of ductal epithelium is infiltrated by lymphocytes, which are also present in the background (Papanicolaou, 20×).

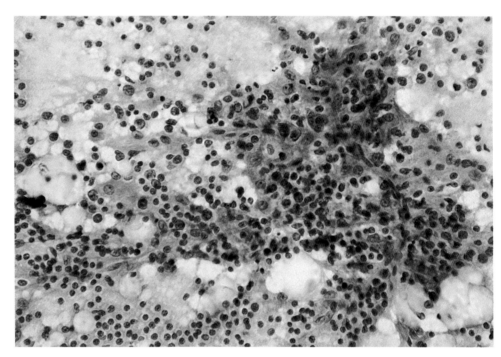

chronic pancreatitis may indeed be so if aspirated during an active, inflammatory phase (Figure 5-15). The cellular components that comprise the hypercellularity are important. A sample of pure ductal-type epithelium should be viewed with suspicion, regardless of bland cytomorphology, because well-differentiated adenocarcinoma may have minimal cytologic changes [7, 8]. An indeterminate mass in a case of chronic active pancreatitis should demonstrate at least an inflammatory cell com-

ponent (see Figures 5-15 and 5-16) or fibrous tissue fragments (Figure 5-17). Multinucleated giant cells may rarely be seen (Figure 5-18). Ductal epithelial cells predominate. The presence of acinar cells (Figure 5-19) depends on the degree of atrophy and fibrosis. At times, the ductal epithelium shows no atypia (Figure 5-20), and the presence of inflammation and fibrosis makes the diagnosis relatively straightforward. Most of the time, however, there is some atypia, which raises the differen-

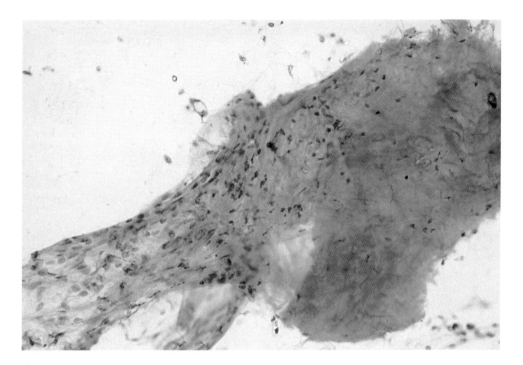

FIGURE 5-17. Chronic pancreatitis. Fragment of dense fibrous tissue associated with little inflammation in a late-stage chronic pancreatitis (Papanicolaou, 10×).

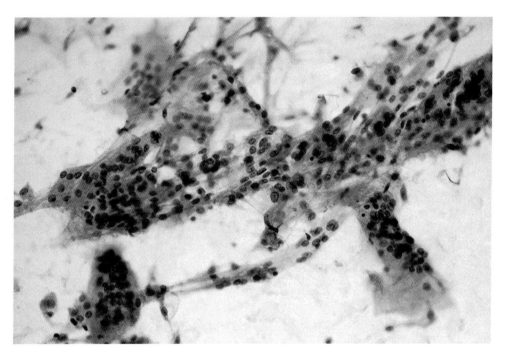

FIGURE 5-18. Chronic pancreatitis. Multinucleated giant cells may be seen in rare cases (Hematoxylin and Eosin, 16×).

FIGURE 5-19. Chronic pancreatitis. Residual acinar cells with reactive nuclear changes associated with a neutrophil (*arrow*) (May-Grünwald–Giemsa, 40×).

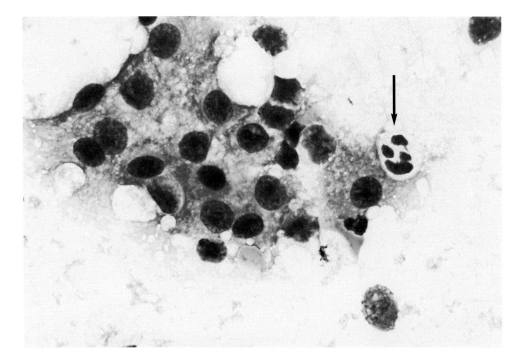

FIGURE 5-20. Chronic pancreatitis. A sheet of normal ductal epithelium with the typical honeycomb appearance and no atypia, and inflammatory cells in the background (Papanicolaou, 20×).

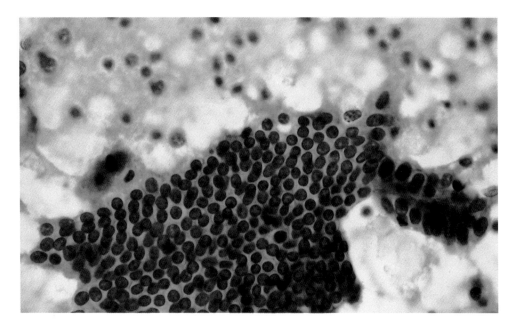

tial diagnosis of adenocarcinoma, one of the most challenging distinctions to be made on FNAB of the pancreas.

The difficulties in the distinction between reactive changes in pancreatitis and adenocarcinoma fall into two categories: (1) markedly atypical reactive ductal changes that appear malignant and (2) well-differentiated adenocarcinoma that appears benign.

Reactive changes in ductal epithelium include squamous metaplasia and reparative, regenerative, and proliferating atypia. In addition to inflammation, previous procedures, instrumentation, and particularly the placement of intraductal stents are culprits in the etiology of reactive atypia. Tremendous caution must be used in the interpretation of atypia in smears with this clinical history. Squamous metaplasia, in the experience at this institution, is rare in both reactive processes and malignancy. The features that define squamous metaplasia of glandular epithelium in general also apply to the pancreatic ductal epithelium. The typical monolayered honeycomb pattern of glandular epithelium is replaced by cells with

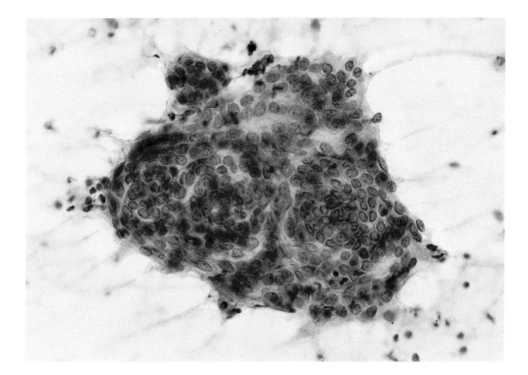

FIGURE 5-21. Chronic pancreatitis. Squamous metaplasia of ductal epithelium demonstrating a common swirling "squamous eddy" pattern (Hematoxylin and Eosin, 20×).

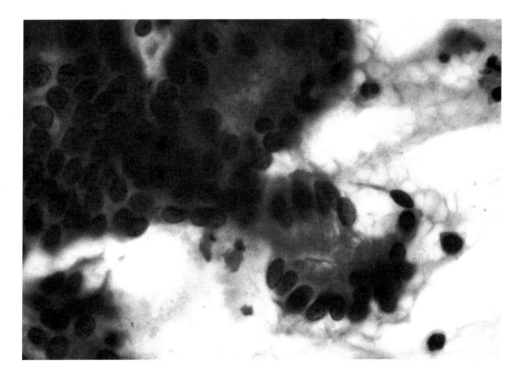

FIGURE 5-22. Chronic pancreatitis. Architectural atypia of ductal epithelium with pseudocribriforming (Papanicolaou, 63×). (Courtesy of Dr. William Frable, Virginia Commonwealth University/Medical College of Virginia School of Medicine, Richmond, VA.)

denser cytoplasm and well-defined borders that may swirl in a squamous eddy (Figure 5-21). The nuclei are uniform and round to oval, with fine chromatin and occasionally prominent nucleoli.

The reactive atypia in the ductal epithelium may be architectural, cytologic, or both. Architectural atypia is the presence of hyperplasia (hypercellular sheets) and pseudocribriforming (Figure 5-22). The nuclei still main-

tain order, polarity, and relative uniformity. Cytologic atypia may be mild, with slight nuclear pleomorphism and cytoplasmic vacuolization (Figure 5-23), moderate with increased nuclear crowding and overlapping (Figure 5-24), or severe with nuclear membrane irregularities and prominent nucleoli (Figure 5-25). Architectural and cytologic atypia may also be present in the same group (Figure 5-26).

FIGURE 5-23. Chronic pancreatitis. Mild cytologic atypia, mild nuclear pleomorphism, and cytoplasmic vacuolization (Papanicolaou, 63×).

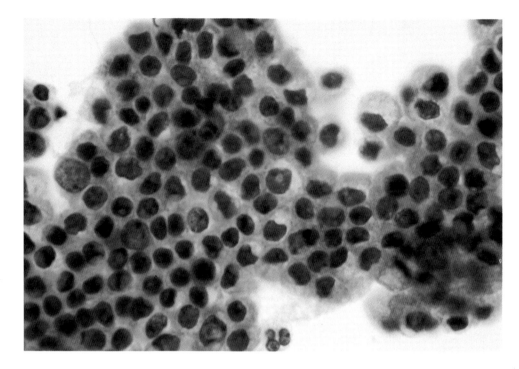

FIGURE 5-24. Chronic pancreatitis. Moderate cytologic atypia with increased nuclear crowding, pleomorphism, and hyperchromasia (Papanicolaou, 63×).

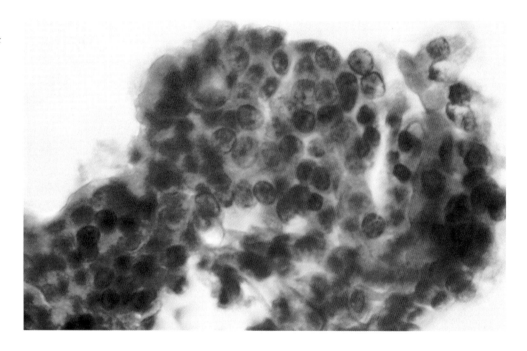

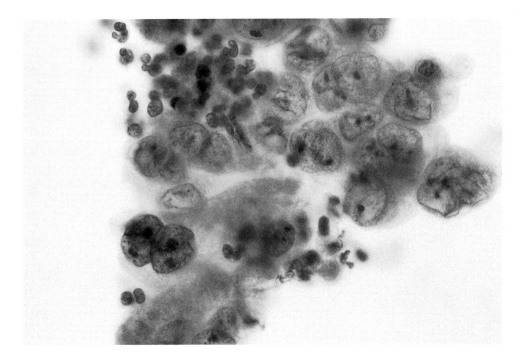

FIGURE 5-25. Chronic pancreatitis. Severe cytologic atypia with marked nuclear membrane irregularities and prominent nucleoli. Note the infiltration of neutrophils into the cluster and the maintenance of cohesion (Papanicolaou, 100×). (Courtesy of Dr. William Frable, Virginia Commonwealth University/Medical College of Virginia School of Medicine, Richmond, VA.)

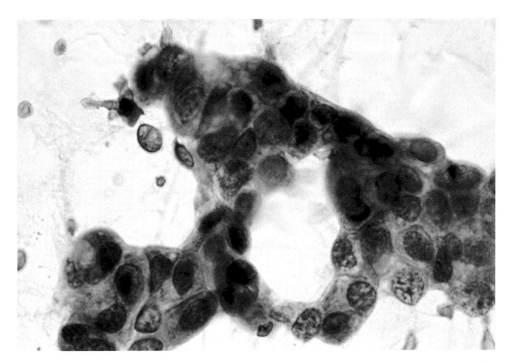

FIGURE 5-26. Chronic pancreatitis. Ductal epithelium demonstrating both architectural and moderate cytologic atypia (Papanicolaou, 63×).

The primary features that distinguish markedly atypical reactive changes from high-grade adenocarcinoma are outlined in Table 5-1. An example of moderately differentiated adenocarcinoma is presented in Figure 5-27 for comparison. Reactive groups are cohesive and without the degree of anisonucleosis, hyperchromasia, nuclear membrane abnormalities, or elevated nuclear-to-cytoplasmic ratio of high-grade carcinoma (see Figure 5-27). Mitoses, necrosis, and intact single epithelial cells are generally not features of reactive ductal changes and are common in adenocarcinoma (see Chapter 7). As such, false-positive diagnoses are generally not the problem: FNAB has a relatively low sensitivity but high specificity in the diagnosis of pancreatic

TABLE 5-1. Distinguishing Cytologic Features of Marked Cellular Atypia in Chronic Pancreatitis and High-Grade Adenocarcinoma

Chronic Pancreatitis	*High-Grade Adenocarcinoma*
Cohesive ductal groups	Dyshesive ductal groups and single intact epithelial cells
Monolayered sheets with focal, mild crowding	Sheets and three-dimensional clusters with marked nuclear crowding and overlapping
No significant nuclear membrane irregularities	Consistent significant nuclear membranes with notching, grooves, and folds
Euchromatic to slightly hyperchromatic nuclei	Marked nuclear hyperchromasia
Normal to slightly increased nuclear-to-cytoplasmic ratio	Consistently increased nuclear-to-cytoplasmic ratio
Minimal nuclear pleomorphism	Marked nuclear pleomorphism
Rare mitoses	Increased mitoses
No necrosis	Frequent necrosis

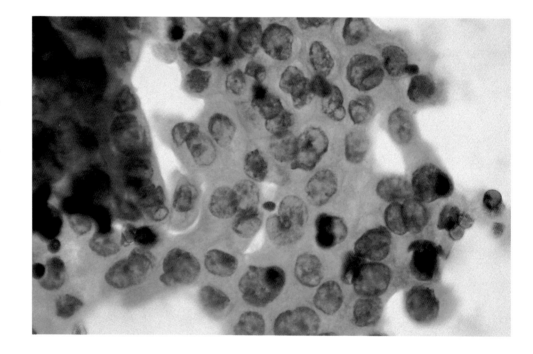

FIGURE 5-27. Moderately differentiated pancreatic adenocarcinoma. Note the severe nuclear membrane abnormalities, nuclear grooves, notches, crowding, and overlapping (Papanicolaou, 100×). (Courtesy of Dr. William Frable, Virginia Commonwealth University/Medical College of Virginia School of Medicine, Richmond, VA.)

adenocarcinoma. Rather, it is the underdiagnosis of well-differentiated adenocarcinoma as reactive epithelial changes that is problematic [9].

Well-differentiated adenocarcinoma of the pancreas lacks obvious cytologic features of malignancy, and because FNAB is unable to determine invasiveness, a feature often relied on in histopathology to make the diagnosis, cytopathologists are extremely conservative in making an unequivocal diagnosis based on smears alone. As such, the use of cell block preparations is a very important adjunct in FNAB of the pancreas. Observing bland-appearing glandular cells (Figure 5-28) infiltrating a sclerotic stroma or surrounding nerves is highly supportive of a diagnosis of malignancy (Figure 5-29). Aspirate smears may be paucicellular due to sclerosis, but cellularity is generally high [8, 9], and the bland-appearing sheets of glandular epithelium are present in a disproportionate amount relative to acini or islet cells [8]. To distinguish such groups from benign ductal groups of the pancreas or intestinal epithelium, one must rely on close, careful inspection of the cells making up the sheets, particularly nuclear detail. These features are outlined in Table 5-2 and include nuclear pleomorphism (Figure 5-30) [10], nuclear enlargement (Figure 5-31) [10, 11], nuclear crowding and overlapping (Figure 5-32) [9], and single intact epithelial cells (Figure 5-33) [11]. Although more

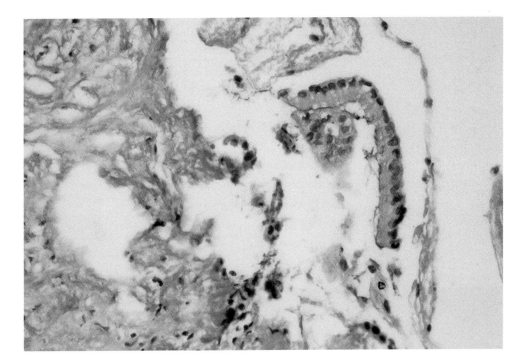

FIGURE 5-28. Well-differentiated adenocarcinoma. Cell block preparation demonstrating strip of extremely benign-appearing glandular epithelium (Hematoxylin and Eosin, 10×).

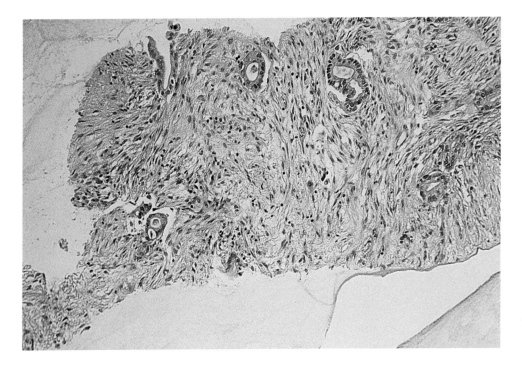

FIGURE 5-29. Well-differentiated adenocarcinoma. Cell block preparation with core biopsy tissue showing infiltration of sclerotic stroma by benign-appearing but malignant glands (Hematoxylin and Eosin, 10×).

TABLE 5-2. Distinguishing Features of Normal and Slightly Reactive Ductal Epithelium in Chronic Pancreatitis and Well-Differentiated Adenocarcinoma

Normal or Chronic Pancreatitis	*Well-Differentiated Adenocarcinoma*
Various cellular elements: ducts, acini, islets	Ducts
Flat, monolayered sheets with uniformly spaced nuclei	Flat, monolayered sheets with noticeable nuclear crowding and overlapping
Round to oval nuclei	Abnormally shaped nuclei: pyramidal, carrot-shaped
Normal chromatin distribution	Frequent chromatin clearing
Few, small nucleoli	Many prominent nucleoli
Rare to no intact single epithelial cells	Few to many intact epithelial cells
Rare to no mitoses	Rare to no mitoses
No necrosis	Generally no necrosis

FIGURE 5-30. Well-differentiated adenocarcinoma. Mild but noticeable nuclear pleomorphism (Papanicolaou, 40×). (Courtesy of Dr. Celeste Powers, State University of New York Health Science Center, Syracuse, NY.)

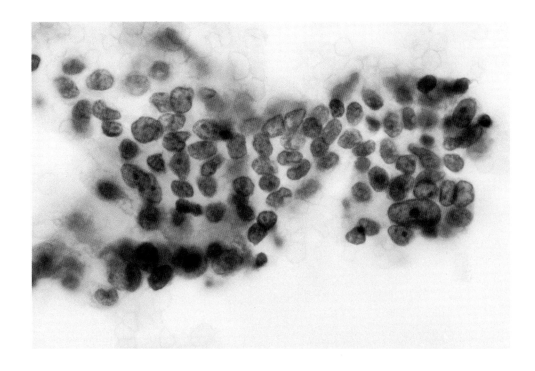

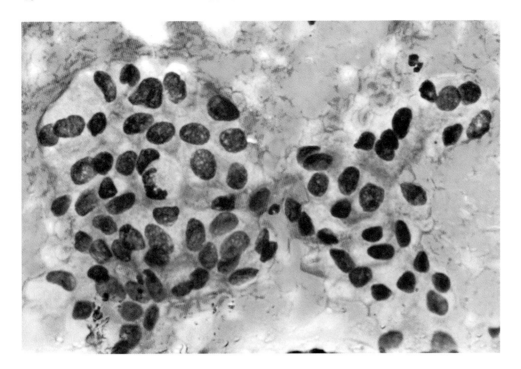

Figure 5-31. Well-differentiated adenocarcinoma. Nuclear enlargement is appreciable when compared with surrounding inflammatory cells or red blood cells (May-Grünwald–Giemsa, 40×; ×1.25 optivar). (Courtesy of Dr. Celeste Powers, State University of New York Health Science Center, Syracuse, NY.)

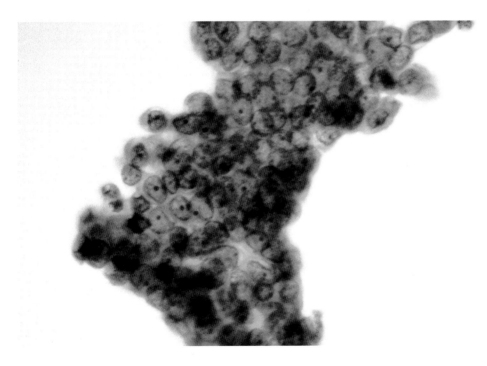

Figure 5-32. Well-differentiated adenocarcinoma. A noticeable increase in nuclear crowding and overlapping is present (Papanicolaou, 40×).

subtle in well-differentiated adenocarcinoma than in higher-grade tumors, these features are present on careful inspection.

Apparent crowding of folded benign sheets of glandular epithelium (Figure 5-34) can be distinguished from true crowding and overlapping by examination of the flat, monolayered portions of the sheets.

Nuclear molding and nuclear membrane irregularities lead to abnormally shaped cells, such as pyramidal and carrot-shaped cells (Figure 5-35) [9]. Also, the chro-

matin in well-differentiated adenocarcinoma more often displays a patchy chromatin clearing rather than hyperchromatism, as in higher-grade tumors (Figure 5-36) [9], a feature best appreciated on alcohol fixed smear.

The minimum diagnostic criteria for the diagnosis of adenocarcinoma established in one series [9] included the presence of two or more of the following major criteria—(1) nuclear crowding or overlapping, (2) irregular nuclear membranes, or (3) irregular chromatin—or one major criterion and three of the fol-

FIGURE 5-33. Well-differentiated adenocarcinoma. Cellular sheet of ductal epithelium with increased nuclear crowding, overlapping, and dyshesiveness producing intact epithelial cells (Papanicolaou, 40×; ×1.25 optivar).

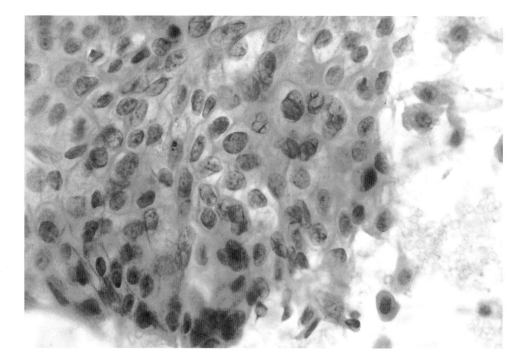

FIGURE 5-34. Chronic pancreatitis with folding of benign ductal sheets giving the appearance of nuclear crowding (Papanicolaou, 40×).

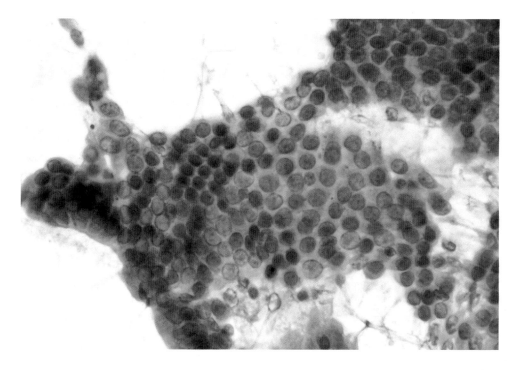

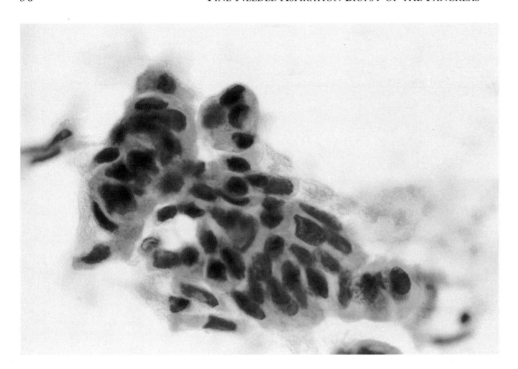

FIGURE 5-35. Well-differentiated adenocarcinoma. Abnormally shaped cells, such as pyramidal and carrot-shaped cells, are produced from crowding, nuclear molding, and nuclear membrane abnormalities (Papanicolaou, 40×).

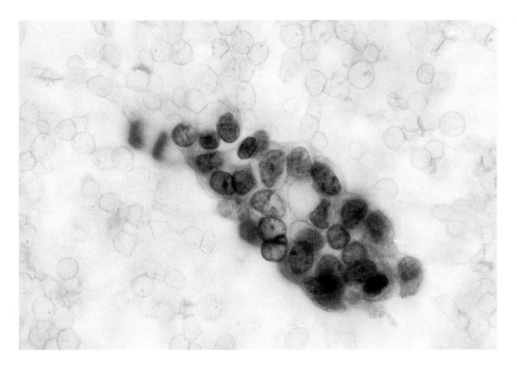

FIGURE 5-36. Well-differentiated adenocarcinoma. Frequent nuclear clearing is displayed rather than hyperchromatism in many well-differentiated tumors (Papanicolaou, 40×). (Courtesy of Dr. Celeste Powers, State University of New York Health Science Center, Syracuse, NY.)

TABLE 5-3. Major and Minor Criteria for the Diagnosis of Adenocarcinoma

Major	Minor
Nuclear crowding or overlapping	Nuclear enlargement
Irregular nuclear membranes	Single epithelial cells
Irregular chromatin	Necrosis
	Mitoses

Source: Excerpted with permission from DB Robins, RL Katz, DB Evans, et al. Fine needle aspiration of the pancreas. In quest of accuracy. Acta Cytol 1995;39:1.

lowing minor criteria—(1) nuclear enlargement (2.5× red blood cells), (2) single epithelial cells, (3) necrosis, (4) mitosis. Using these criteria, the diagnostic precision was 100% (Table 5-3).

Cytologic Features of Chronic Pancreatitis
- Mixed cellular elements: ducts, acini, inflammation, fibrosis
- Cellular but cohesive ductal groups
- Normal to slightly increased nuclear-to-cytoplasmic ratio
- Minimal nuclear pleomorphism
- Euchromatic to slightly hyperchromatic nuclei
- No significant nuclear membrane abnormalities
- Rare mitoses; no necrosis

REFERENCES

1. DelMaschio A, Vanzulli A, Sironi S, et al. Pancreatic cancer versus chronic pancreatitis: diagnosis with CA19-9 assessment, US, CT, and CT-guided fine-needle biopsy. Radiology 1991;178:95.

2. Luetmer PH, Stephens DH, Ward EM. Chronic pancreatitis: reassessment with current CT. Radiology 1989;171:353.

3. Cruickshank AH. Pathology of the Pancreas. Berlin: Springer-Verlag, 1986.

4. VanDyke JA, Stanley RJ, Berland LL. Pancreatic imaging. Ann Intern Med 1985;102:212.

5. Fishman EK, Jones B, Siegelman SS. The Indeterminate Pancreatic Mass: Carcinoma Versus Focal Pancreatitis. In SS Siegelman (ed), Computed Tomography of the Pancreas. New York: Churchill Livingstone, 1983;157.

6. Cotran RS, Kumar V, Robbins SL. Pathologic Basis of Disease (5th ed). Philadelphia: Saunders, 1994.

7. Saez A, Catala I, Brossa R, et al. Intraoperative fine needle aspiration cytology of pancreatic lesions. A study of 90 cases. Acta Cytol 1995;39:485.

8. Hejka AG, Bernacki EG. Cytopathology of well-differentiated columnar adenocarcinoma of the pancreas diagnosed by fine needle aspiration. Acta Cytol 1990;34:716.

9. Robins DB, Katz RL, Evans DB, et al. Fine needle aspiration of the pancreas. In quest of accuracy. Acta Cytol 1995;39:1.

10. Cohen MB, Egerter DP, Holly EA, et al. Pancreatic adenocarcinoma: regression analysis to identify improved cytologic criteria. Diagn Cytopathol 1991;7:341.

11. Francillon YJ, Bagby J, Abreo F, Turbat-Herrera E. Criteria for predicting malignancy in fine needle aspiration biopsies (FNAB) of the pancreas and biliary tree. Acta Cytologica 1996;40:1084.

Cystic Lesions

Barbara A. Centeno

The differential diagnosis of pancreatic cystic lesions is varied; cystic lesions can be classified as congenital, inflammatory, and neoplastic (Table 6-1). The vast majority are pseudocysts, which account for approximately 75–90% [1–3] of all pancreatic cystic lesions. Cystic neoplasms, which account for approximately 5% of all tumors of the pancreas [4], include serous cystadenoma (SCA), mucinous cystic neoplasm (MCN), mucinous cystadenocarcinoma (MCA), and solid pseudopapillary tumor (SPPT); congenital cysts, infections, cysts, and other rare entities constitute the remainder.

WHY SHOULD PANCREATIC CYST FLUIDS BE EVALUATED?

The preoperative diagnosis of pancreatic cysts using clinical or radiologic criteria is not always specific for the distinction of neoplasms from inflammatory cysts and benign from malignant neoplasms [3]. Over a 12-year span, more than one-third of patients referred to the Massachusetts General Hospital (MGH) with cystic neoplasms were misdiagnosed as having pseudocysts [3], and the literature contains numerous reports of cystic neoplasms misdiagnosed as pseudocysts [2, 5–7]. Misdiagnosis has led to inappropriate therapy and fatal results for some patients.

Errors also occur on frozen sections and on permanent sections due to variability of the cyst lining and epithelial denudation [3]. One study reported that 20% of all cystic neoplasms were incorrectly classified by frozen section analysis [8].

Appropriate preoperative diagnosis is essential to planning surgical management. Pseudocysts may be treated by observation or in situ drainage. SCA may be observed when asymptomatic. Most other neoplasms, including MCN, SPPT, and cystic pancreatic endocrine tumors, require surgical resection because all are potentially malignant [3].

Analysis of the pancreatic cyst fluids for cytology, pancreatic enzymes, tumor marker levels, and viscosity has gained recognition within recent years as a potential means of diagnosing pancreatic cystic lesions preoperatively.

NON-NEOPLASTIC CYSTS

Pseudocysts

Pseudocysts are the most common cystic lesions of the pancreas, accounting for 75–90% of all cases [1–3]. They follow bouts of acute pancreatitis, acute exacerbations of chronic pancreatitis, trauma, or surgery. They result when ducts rupture, spilling the digestive juices into the lesser sac, causing an inflammatory response that walls off semidigested and necrotic material [1, 9]. Congenital pancreatic pseudocysts have been reported [10], and multiple pseudocysts may also occur [11]. Typically, pseudocysts present as a unilocular cyst that, depending on the type of pseudocyst, may or may not connect with the pancreatic duct as demonstrated by endoscopic retrograde cholangiopancreatography (ERCP) [12]. Resection specimens show a unilocular cyst usually filled with blood and fibrin (Figure 6-1). Histologically, they are characterized by a fibrous cyst wall with variable amounts of inflammation and granulation tissue in earlier lesions. No cyst lining is seen (Figure 6-2). The cyst lumen may contain blood, fibrin, and inflammation [1].

Table 6-1. Classification of Cysts of the Pancreas

Congenital cysts	Infectious cysts
Simple or solitary true cyst	Secondary pancreatic infections
Polycystic diseases	Hydatid cysts
Cystic fibrosis	*Giardia*
Enteric duplication cysts	Cystic neoplasms
Biliary and pancreatic duct anomalies	Serous cystadenoma
Dermoid cyst (is also classified as neoplasm)	Mucinous cystic neoplasm
Lymphoepithelial cyst	Mucinous cystadenocarcinoma
Pseudocyst	Vascular
Postinflammatory	Lymphangioma
Post-traumatic	Hemangioma
Postsurgical	Solid pseudopapillary tumor
Congenital	Cystic pancreatic endocrine tumor
Retention cyst	Acinar cell cystadenocarcinoma
Postobstuctive due to pancreatic cancer, pancreatic lithiasis,	Ductal carcinoma with cystic degeneration
or chronic pancreatitis	Any neoplasm with cystic degeneration
Cholelithiasis and cholecystitis	Miscellaneous cysts
Parasitic infections obstructing ducts such as amebic,	Nutritional (tropical) fibrocalcific pancreatitis
Clonorchis sinensis, Ascaris lumbricoides	Extrapancreatic cysts

Aspiration of a pseudocyst usually obtains a generous amount of turbid, red-brown or brown fluid. The cytology is characterized by a variable inflammatory component, including neutrophils and histiocytes, granular background debris, fibrin, blood (Figure 6-3), and occasionally bile pigment (Figure 6-4). Hemosiderin-laden macrophages may be numerous (Figure 6-5). Cyst-lining epithelial cells are not found; however, normal pancreatic epithelium, metaplastic epithelium (Figure 6-6), mesothelial cells, or fibroblasts may be inadvertently aspirated [13].

Cytology of Pseudocysts

- Variable inflammatory cell component
- Hemosiderin-laden macrophages
- Blood, granular debris, and occasionally bile pigment in background
- No cyst-lining epithelium
- ± Normal pancreatic components and fibroblasts

The differential diagnosis includes secondary pancreatic infections, to be discussed further in that section, and cystic neoplasms (Table 6-2). Epithelium from normal structures may be inadvertently obtained during the procedure, but the presence of mucinous epithelium that is not a contaminant should be addressed. The presence of background mucin, mucin-containing histiocytes, or both, even in the absence of mucinous epithelium, excludes the diagnosis of pseudocyst and should lead the observer to search for evidence of a mucinous neoplasm [13, 14].

Retention Cysts

Retention cysts are intraparenchymal, occurring secondary to obstruction of the pancreatic duct system from a number of causes, including obstructing cancer, chronic pancreatitis, or parasitic infections [1]. Retention cysts also result from tropical or malnutritional fibrocalcific pancreatitis, occurring secondary to protein malnutrition or alcoholism [15, 16]. Because retention cysts result from distortion and dilation of the pancreatic duct, ERCP demonstrates an intraparenchymal cyst that connects with the pancreatic ductal system. The cyst wall is reportedly lined with ductal epithelium [1], but inflammation, pressure of the cyst contents, and necrosis may destroy the lining. The immediately adjacent parenchyma usually shows

FIGURE 6-1. Cross section of a pseudocyst resection. *C* marks the cyst cavity, which is lined by hemorrhagic, friable tissue. *P* marks the surrounding soft tissue and pancreatic parenchyma.

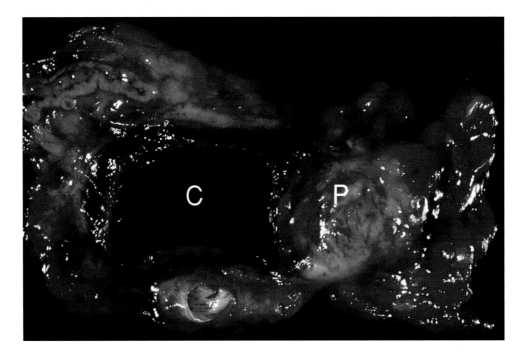

FIGURE 6-2. Biopsy of pseudocyst. The wall is fibrotic with a lymphoplasmacytic and histiocytic infiltrate. Notice the absence of an epithelial lining (Hematoxylin and Eosin, 20×).

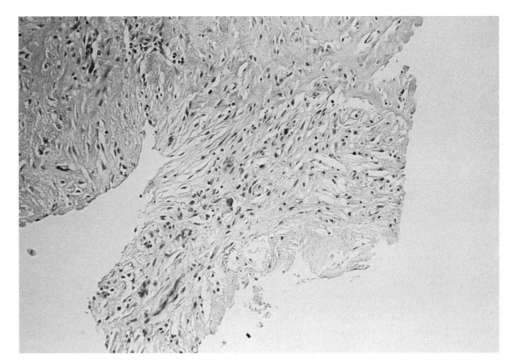

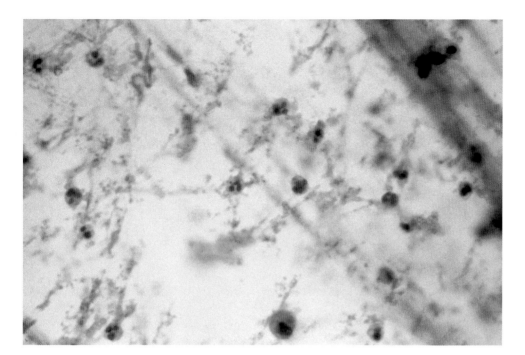

FIGURE 6-3. Pseudocyst. Few neutrophils and histiocytes in fibrin and granular debris (Papanicolaou, 40×; ×1.25 optivar).

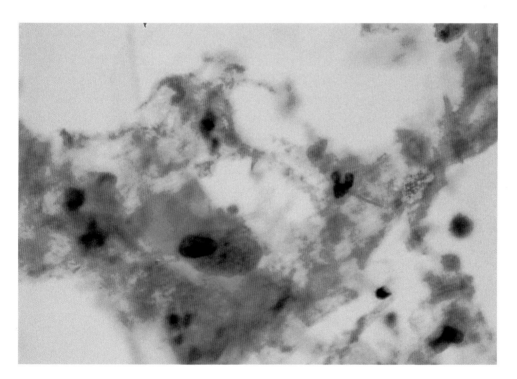

FIGURE 6-4. Pseudocyst. Histiocytes, granular debris, and golden-yellow bile pigment (Papanicolaou, 40×).

FIGURE 6-5. Pseudocyst.
Hemosiderin-laden
macrophages (Papanico-
laou, 40×; ×1.25 optivar).

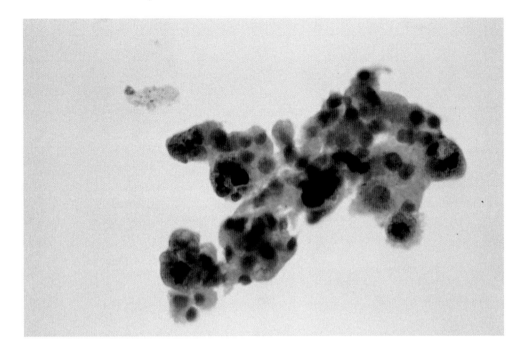

FIGURE 6-6. Pseudocyst.
Keratinized squamous cells
present, consistent with
squamous metaplasia aris-
ing in an adjacent duct
(Papanicolaou, 40×).

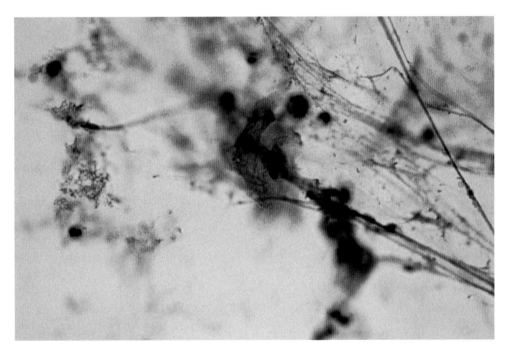

Table 6-2. Cytologic Differential Diagnosis of Pancreatic Cystic Lesions

Lesion	Location	Age, Sex	Cytology
Pseudocyst	Extrapancreatic	Variable	Granular debris and fibrin Inflammatory cells and hemosiderin laden macrophages No cyst-lining epithelial cells ± Contaminants
Abscess	Intrapancreatic	Variable	Neutrophilic infiltrate with a proteinaceous background Culture positive
Lymphoepithelial cyst	Lesser sac	Adults, males	Anucleated and nucleated benign squames Keratinous debris and cholesterol crystal ± Lymphocytes
Vascular tumors	Varies	Adults	Spindle-shaped endothelial cells in sheets or singly Smooth muscle
Cystic pancreatic endocrine tumor	Variable	Adults	Monomorphic, dyshesive Salt-and-pepper chromatin Plasmacytoid occasionally Neuroendocrine differentiation on immunocytochemical studies and electron microscopy
Solid pseudopapillary tumor	Tail (most commonly)	Teens to 30 yrs (almost always female)	Cellular Branching fragments with central fibrovascular cores having a mucinous stroma Bland cells with scant cytoplasm Balls of myxoid stroma the hallmark
Serous cystadenoma	Tail	Elderly	Monomorphic cuboidal epithelial cells in flat sheets and groups Glycogen in cytoplasm No mucin
Mucinous cystic neoplasms	Tail, body	Middle-aged females	Background mucin and columnar epithelium Absence of malignant nuclear features, necrosis, and mitoses
Mucinous cystadenocarcinoma	Tail, body	Middle-aged females	Mucinous epithelium in papillary groups, three-dimensional groups, or as signet-ring cells Cytomorphologic features of malignancy Necrosis and mitoses
Ductal adenocarcinoma with cystic degeneration	Head	Older than 40 yrs, males	Adenocarcinoma Cystic or necrotic debris in the background

changes of chronic pancreatitis with fibrosis, islet cells, and atrophy of the parenchyma. The reported cytomorphology reflects these features and is characterized by inflammatory cells, islet cells from the wall, and some ductal epithelium [17].

Cytology of Retention Cysts

- Variable inflammatory component
- ± Ductal epithelial cells
- Islet cells from adjacent parenchyma

The differential diagnosis includes pseudocyst, because the cytologic features of the two may overlap, and MCN, because theoretically retention cysts may contain mucinous epithelium or background mucin originating from the pancreatic ductal epithelium. However, retention cysts are small and relatively uncommon [1], with the characteristic ERCP finding of a cyst in continuity with a strictured or obstructed pancreatic ductal system, and therefore are unlikely to present a diagnostic dilemma. The distinction from MCN is discussed in that section.

FIGURE 6-7. Abscess, fungal. Fine needle aspiration biopsy smears show branching pseudohyphae (*arrow*) consistent with *Candida albicans*; species was confirmed by fungal culture (Papanicolaou, 40×; ×1.6 optivar).

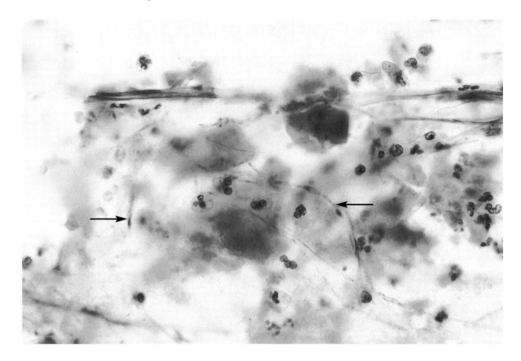

Infectious Cysts

Secondary Pancreatic Infections

Secondary pancreatic infections, which may occasionally appear as pancreatic cysts radiologically, can be classified as infected pseudocysts, pancreatic abscesses appearing as walled-off material in the lesser sac after acute pancreatitis or trauma, or infected pancreatic necrosis [18]. The presentation and therapy are distinct from an uninfected pseudocyst [19]. Bacterial organisms are cultured more than 90% of the time and are most often enteric [19], but some have resulted from infection with *Candida albicans* (Figure 6-7) [20]. Prognosis depends on the type of clinical entity. Infected pseudocysts are associated with the least morbidity, infected necrosis is associated with the most, and pancreatic abscesses demonstrate an intermediate prognosis [18].

The fine needle aspiration biopsy (FNAB) specimen is characterized by an abundance of neutrophils, with nuclear debris and proteinaceous background material that is not readily evident on ThinPrep smears (Figures 6-8 and 6-9). Cultures will grow infectious organisms in most cases. Secondary pancreatic infections can be distinguished from an uncomplicated pseudocyst by the nature of the inflammatory response, the background proteinaceous debris, and the culture results [21].

Cytology of Secondary Pancreatic Cysts

- Numerous neutrophils
- Proteinaceous background
- Cultures positive
- Organisms present by culture

Helminthic and Protozoal Infections

A number of helminths may infect the pancreatic ducts, causing duct obstruction [1]. Hydatid cysts may rarely develop in the pancreas and cause obstructive jaundice [22–24] or present as an abdominal mass [23]. The diagnosis may be suggested clinically by the epidemiologic setting, cyst wall calcifications, daughter cysts demonstrated on ultrasound, peripheral eosinophilia, and positive hydatid serology [25].

Aspiration of a hydatid cyst is reportedly safe and sensitive [26, 27]. Hooklets and protoscolices are diagnostic. In one case report, however, aspiration of the cyst fluid yielded clear fluid with a low amylase content, no malignant cells, and no hooklets or protoscolices [22]. In a situation such as this, other clinical findings and cyst fluid parameters are necessary for the diagnosis.

Cytology of Hydatid Cyst

- Hooklets
- Protoscolices

Giardia has also been detected in pancreatic cyst fluid (Figure 6-10) (personal experience, unpublished data). One report described numerous pancreatic cysts containing *Giardia* in a diabetic patient [28]. Care must be taken to ensure that such an infectious agent is not a contaminant from the gastrointestinal tract.

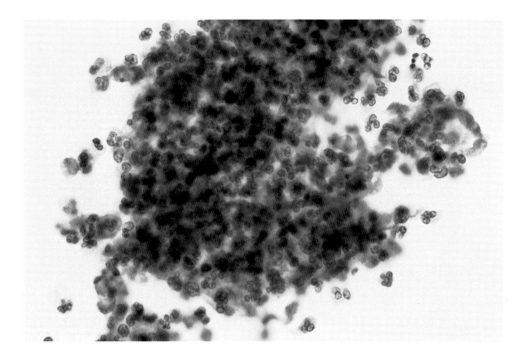

FIGURE 6-8. Abscess. Thick collection of inflammatory cells, embedded in proteinaceous material (Papanicolaou, 40×; ×1.6 optivar).

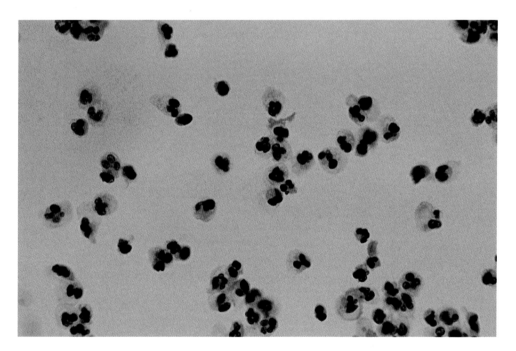

FIGURE 6-9. Abscess. The inflammatory infiltrate of the abscess seen in Figure 6-7 is composed of neutrophils (Papanicolaou, 40×; ×1.6 optivar).

FIGURE 6-10. *Giardia.* Aspiration of a solitary, 0.9-cm cyst in the head of the pancreas yielded numerous *Giardia.* The organisms are pear shaped and binucleated (Papanicolaou, 100×; ×1.6 optivar).

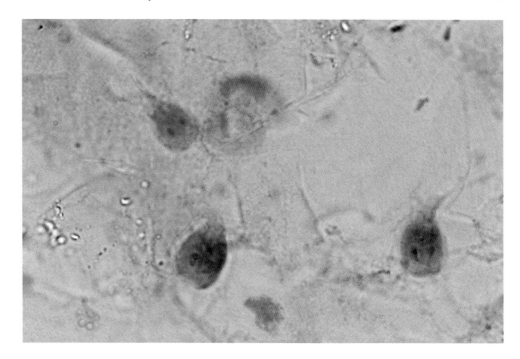

Congenital Cysts

Congenital cysts are more often single than multiple, unilocular than multilocular, and more frequently located in the pancreatic body or tail than in the head [29, 30]. The most common type is the simple cyst or solitary true cyst, most frequently found in children within the first few years of life but also rarely reported in adults [31, 32]. Single cysts are infrequently of clinical significance [30, 31], but they may present with abdominal distention, vomiting, or jaundice, or as an asymptomatic abdominal mass [29]. They are believed to result from anomalous development of the pancreatic ductal system wherein sequestered segments of a primitive secretory ductal system give rise to a cystic lesion [33]. A female predominance has been noted [29]. Grossly, they appear as cysts with thin walls containing clear, serous fluid. No connection with the ductal system is seen [31]. A flattened, single layer of cuboidal epithelium with bland nuclei lines the cysts, and the wall is composed of dense fibrous tissue (Figure 6-11). Experience with cyst fluid analysis of these lesions is limited. Studies of cyst fluid pancreatic enzyme levels have been contradictory, reportedly elevated in some cases [34], but low or within normal levels in others [31, 32, 35, 36]; among the tumor markers, carcinoembryonic antigen (CEA) has been reported within normal levels [31, 32], and CA 19-9 and CA 125 levels have been elevated [31].

Experience with cytologic examination of fluid from congenital cysts is equally limited. Sperti et al. [31] reported an acellular sample. Other authors reported benign epithelial cells [35] but did not elaborate on their cytomorphologic features. Frias-Hidvegi described a scantly cellular sample with normal epithelial cells, occasionally in monolayers, mimicking a reactive process, with abundant, cyanophilic, delicate cytoplasm and fine, evenly distributed chromatin and multinucleated, reactive-appearing single cells in a congenital cyst from a patient with von Hippel–Lindau syndrome [17]. Aspiration of a simple cyst in our department showed a scantly cellular sample containing single, cuboidal epithelial cells with basophilic, well-defined cytoplasm and round, bland nuclei (Figure 6-12).

Cytology of Simple Cysts

- Scant cellularity, possibly acellular
- Single cells
- Cuboidal shape
- Sharp, cytoplasmic borders
- Basophilic cytoplasm
- Round to oval nuclei with fine chromatin

Aspiration of these cysts is likely to be nondiagnostic because of the scant cellularity. Reliance on other markers will probably be necessary to exclude pseudocyst or cystic neoplasms.

Other congenital or hereditary conditions associated with cysts in the pancreas include polycystic pancreas without related anomalies in other organs [30], pancreatic cysts associated with polycystic renal disease [30], the von Hippel–Lindau syndrome, [30, 37, 38] renal-hepatic-pancreatic dysplasia [39], oral-facial-digital syndrome type I [40], pancreaticobiliary defects [41], and macrocysts from cystic fibrosis [30]. A cystic hamartoma of the pancreas, enteric duplication cysts, and ciliated foregut cysts have also been reported [42–44]. Aspiration of one enteroge-

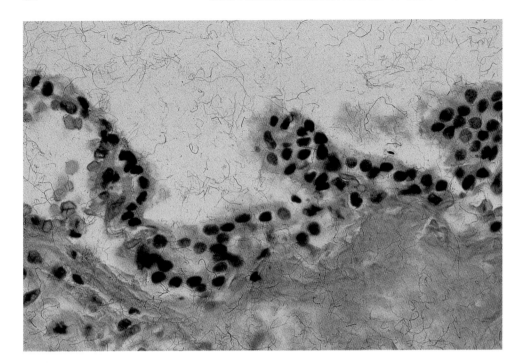

FIGURE 6-11. Simple cyst. The cyst is lined by a single layer of homogeneous, cuboidal epithelium with bland, uniform nuclei and slightly eosinophilic cytoplasm, which is thrown into folds. The wall is densely fibrotic (Hematoxylin and Eosin, 40×; ×1.25 optivar).

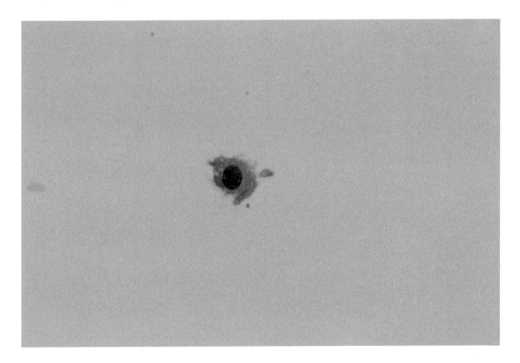

FIGURE 6-12. Simple cyst. Scantly cellular specimen composed of single cells with abundant, well-defined, basophilic cytoplasm and bland, round nuclei (Papanicolaou, 40×; ×1.6 optivar).

FIGURE 6-13. Lymphoepithelial cyst. Resection specimen showing cyst lined by mature squamous epithelium with a granular layer. The cyst cavity contains anucleated squames and cholesterol clefts. A dense lymphocytic infiltrate permeates the wall (Hematoxylin and Eosin, 10×).

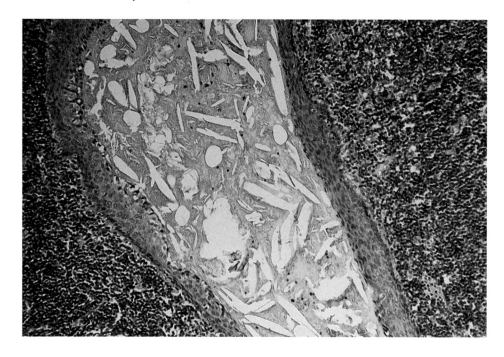

nous duplication cyst produced acellular smears (personal experience, unpublished data). Other cyst fluid analysis showed elevated levels of CEA, CA 125, amylase and a high viscosity, a profile suggestive of MCN [44].

Lymphoepithelial Cyst of the Pancreas

Lymphoepithelial cyst of the pancreas (LECP) is a rare entity; only 26 cases have been reported to the date of this writing [45–49]. We have seen two unreported cases in our department. The male-to-female ratio is 16:3, and patients have ranged from 32 to 73 years in age. Abdominal pain is the most common presenting symptom; other signs and symptoms include nausea and vomiting, malaise, fever, weight loss, fatigue, and diarrhea. A significant percentage are discovered incidentally [45]. At least four different theories about the histogenesis of these cysts have been proposed. The most accepted to date is that a lymphoepithelial cyst arises from a benign epithelial inclusion or ectopic pancreas in a peripancreatic lymph node [45]. Computed tomography (CT) scans display a well-circumscribed, round mass protruding from the anterior surface of the pancreas into the lesser sac. Ultrasonography shows a cystic mass [45].

Grossly, the cyst is always single, well circumscribed, and filled with "cheesy" material [45]. Histologically, the cyst is lined by squamous keratinizing epithelium. The cyst lumen is filled with keratinous debris and cholesterol clefts. Lymphoid tissue with some lymphoid follicles surrounds the cyst lining (Figure 6-13).

Benign superficial squamous cells and anucleated squames are the main finding on FNAB smears; platelike cholesterol crystals, histiocytes, and lymphocytes are additional findings (Figures 6-14 and 6-15) [49–51]. These features contrast with those of lymphoepithelial cysts of the parotid gland, in which lymphocytes are numerous [50]. The cell block shows a fragment of tissue with a squamous lining, a dense lymphocytic infiltrate in the stroma, and keratinous debris in the background (Figure 6-16).

Cytology of Lymphoepithelial Cyst

- Anucleated squames
- Mature, superficial squamous cells
- ± Lymphocytes, histiocytes
- Cholesterol clefts

The differential diagnosis includes the following (see Table 6-2):

- Pseudocyst
- Other squamous-lined cysts, such as dermoid cyst or splenic epidermoid cyst
- Other cystic neoplasms
- Squamous cell carcinoma

The presence of keratinous debris and abundant mature nucleated squamous cells and anucleated squames excludes the diagnosis of pseudocyst. A dermoid cyst typically contains sebaceous material, columnar cells, mesodermal elements, or hair in addition to the squamous component [50, 52]; however, distinction among the various types of squamous cysts that occur in this region may not be possible or clinically relevant. Other cystic neoplasms lack a squamous component. The squamous cells in LECP lack the cytologic features of

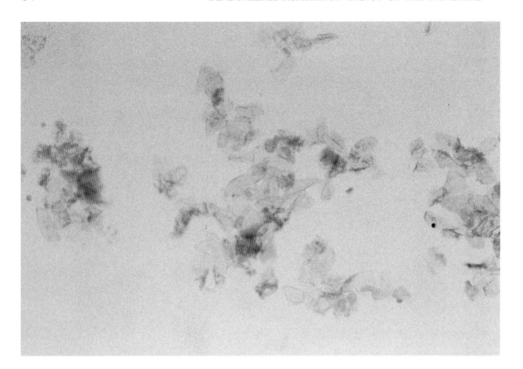

FIGURE 6-14. Lymphoepithelial cyst. Numerous anucleated squames (Papanicolaou, 62.5×). (Courtesy of Dr. James Cappellari, Bowman Gray School of Medicine of Wake Forest University, Winston-Salem, NC.)

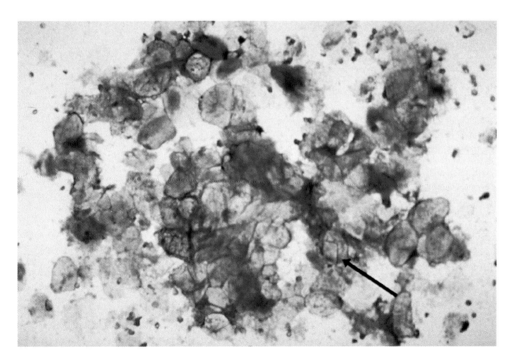

FIGURE 6-15. Lymphoepithelial cyst. Anucleated squames and cholesterol crystals (arrow) (Diff Quik, 62.5×). (Courtesy of Dr. James Cappellari, Bowman Gray School of Medicine of Wake Forest University, Winston-Salem, NC.)

Figure 6-16. Lymphoep-
ithelial cyst. Cell block
specimen showing a frag-
ment of tissue lined by
maturing squamous epithe-
lium, with a dense lymphocytic infiltrate in the wall.
The background contains
keratinous debris (Hema-
toxylin and Eosin, 10×).

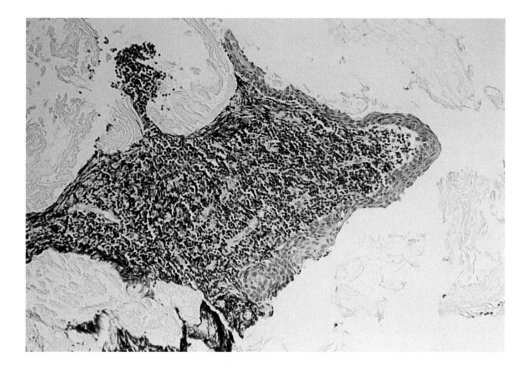

FIGURE 6-17. Dermoid
cyst. Numerous anucleated
squames with keratinous
material (Papanicolaou,
40×; ×1.6 optivar).

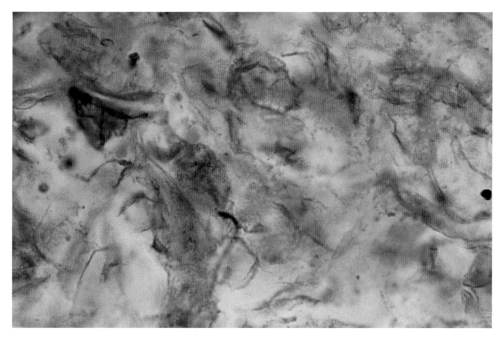

malignancy, excluding the diagnosis of squamous cell
carcinoma.

Dermoid Cysts

Dermoid cysts of the pancreas, also known as *cystic teratomas*, are rare and are believed to develop from a
totipotential cell in an embryonic rest [53, 54]. They are
included in this section because they are in the differential diagnosis of squamous-lined cysts even though they
are neoplasms. They occur mostly in infants, children,
and young adults and show a slight female predominance, in contrast to LECP [54]. Their gross and microscopic features are similar to those of dermoid cysts
occurring at other sites.

FNAB of a dermoid cyst yields turbid, tan cyst
fluid that contains amorphous, sebaceous material; anucleated and nucleated squamous cells; neutrophils; and
keratinous debris. A lymphocytic component may also
be present (Figures 6-17 and 6-18) [52].

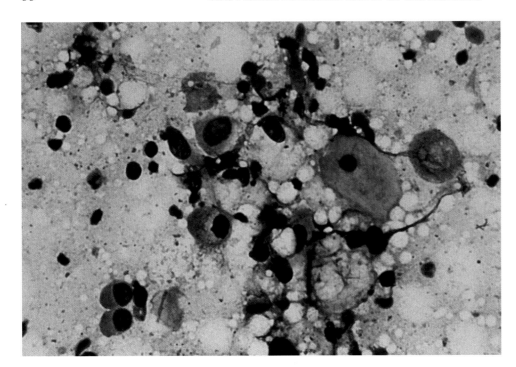

FIGURE 6-18. Dermoid cyst. Squamous cells, anucleated squames, sebaceous background material, and lymphoplasmacytic infiltrate (Diff-Quik, 40×; ×1.6 optivar).

Cytology of Dermoid Cysts

- Amorphous sebaceous material
- Squamous cells
- Anucleated squames
- Inflammation

The differential diagnosis is similar to that for LECP.

Splenic Epidermoid Cyst

A case of splenic epidermoid cyst developing in an accessory spleen in the pancreas has been described [55]. Histologically, these cysts are characterized by a squamous cyst lining with keratinization and a wall composed of splenic parenchyma. Splenic epidermoid cyst is included in the differential diagnosis of squamous-lined cysts occurring in the pancreas or peripancreatic areas.

NEOPLASTIC CYSTS

Serous Cystadenoma (Microcystic Adenoma, Glycogen-Rich Cystadenoma)

SCA of the pancreas is a rare cystic neoplasm defined by Compagno and Oertel in 1978 [56]. SCA typically occurs in elderly patients and has a slight female predilection [56]. Presenting symptoms include abdominal pain, weight loss, and jaundice. Some patients present with an abdominal mass or an incidentally discovered mass on imaging procedures. The classic radiologic picture of a microcystic lesion with a central stellate scar is rarely present, leading to difficulties in the preoperative diagnosis. Small loculations are apparent only 50% of the time [3]; macrocystic variants have been described [57, 58], and the central stellate scar is infrequently found (11% of cases in one study) [3]. SCA are typically benign and indolent [56], but locally aggressive and malignant behavior has been reported [59–62]. Immunohistochemical and electron microscopic studies have shown that the tumor cells resemble centroacinar cells [63].

On gross examination, innumerable small cysts filled with clear fluid impart a honeycombed or spongy appearance to the cut surface, and fibrous bands with or without calcifications form a central stellate scar (Figure 6-19), although not all SCA have this classic appearance. Macrocystic variants have a prominent, large cyst, usually filled with blood (Figure 6-20). Histologically, the tumors are composed of numerous small cysts surrounded by fibrous stroma having a rich capillary network (Figure 6-21) and lined by flattened, cuboidal epithelium with clear cytoplasm and bland homogeneous nuclei (Figure 6-22). Some papillary projections may be seen. Glycogen has been demonstrated in the cells with the use of periodic acid–Schiff (PAS) with and without diastase (Figure 6-23).

The cytology of these neoplasms has been described in a number of series and case reports [13, 64–67]. Smears of these tumors are scantly cellular with a proteinaceous background and blood. The cells are arranged in monolayered sheets and have round, bland, homogeneous nuclei and clear or vacuolated cytoplasm with sharp cyto-

FIGURE 6-19. Serous cystadenoma. Gross photograph demonstrating well-circumscribed tumor mass composed of numerous, small cysts, 0.2–2.0 cm in diameter, with a central stellate scar.

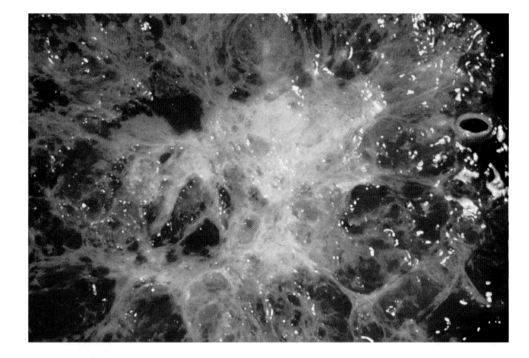

FIGURE 6-20. Serous cystadenoma. Gross photograph of macrocystic serous cystadenoma showing a well-circumscribed neoplasm with a central large cyst containing abundant hemorrhagic, friable material. The tumor parenchyma adjacent to the macrocyst is composed of more typical microcysts. Smaller cysts are seen adjacent to the macrocyst. (Reprinted with permission from Lewandrowski, K et al. Macrocystic cystadenoma of the pancreas: A morphologic variant differing from microcystic adenoma. Hum Pathol. 1992 23:871-875 WB Saunders, Philadephia.)

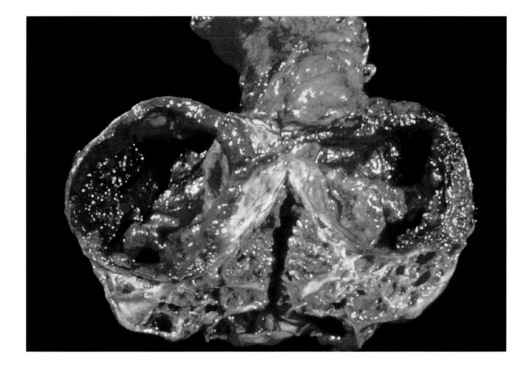

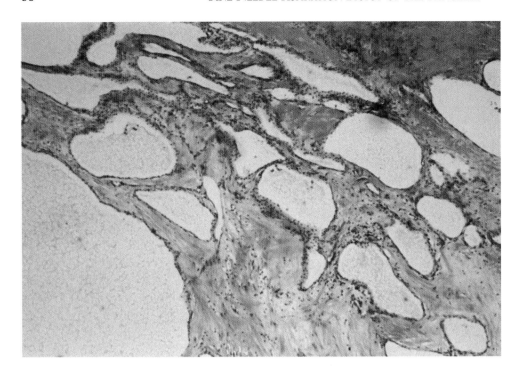

FIGURE 6-21. Serous cystadenoma. Histologically, the neoplasm is composed of numerous microcysts containing clear fluid, surrounded by a dense, fibrous stroma (Hematoxylin and Eosin, 20×).

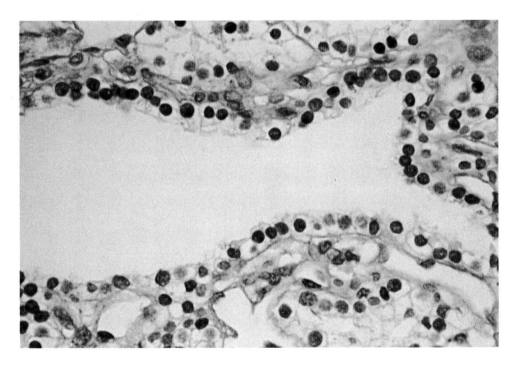

FIGURE 6-22. Serous cystadenoma. High-power view of Figure 6-20 showing the cyst lining, composed of a monolayer of homogeneous, cuboidal epithelium with clear cytoplasm (Hematoxylin and Eosin, 40×).

FIGURE 6-23. Serous cystadenoma. A periodic acid–Schiff (PAS) stain demonstrates the presence of cytoplasmic glycogen that is digested by the diastase reaction (not shown) (PAS, 40×).

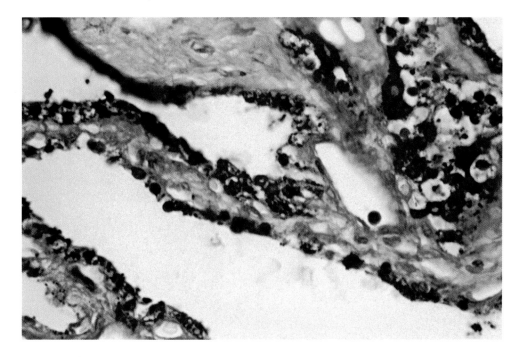

FIGURE 6-24. Serous cystadenoma. Fine needle aspiration biopsy smear showing a scantly cellular specimen with cohesive monolayered sheets of cells. The background contains blood and proteinaceous material (Modified Wright Giemsa, 25×).

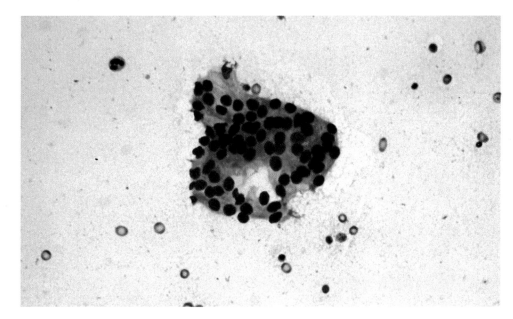

plasmic borders (Figures 6-24 and 6-25). Intracytoplasmic glycogen is demonstrated by the PAS stain with and without diastase digestion (Figure 6-26). ThinPrep smears typically have a clean background. The cells occur in small clusters, the chromatin detail is lost, and small vacuoles are seen in the cytoplasm (Figure 6-27).

Cytology of Serous Cystadenoma

- Scant cellularity
- Watery fluid
- Proteinaceous or bloody background
- Monolayered sheets or small, flat clusters
- Homogenous, bland, round nuclei
- Clear cytoplasm with well-defined borders
- Cytoplasmic glycogen demonstrated by PAS with and without diastase

Problems in interpretation occur because of the scant cellularity, which may lead to a nondiagnostic interpretation. Most aspirates of these lesions lack epithelial groups and are frequently nondiagnostic [13, 14]. The differential diagnosis includes the following (see also Table 6-2):

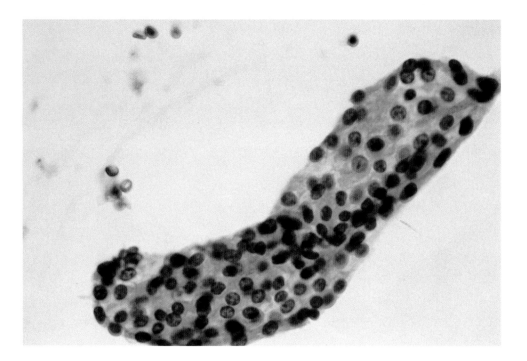

FIGURE 6-25. Serous cystadenoma. Fine needle aspiration biopsy smear showing a monolayered sheet of cells. The cytoplasm is well-defined, cuboidal, and basophilic but finely granular. The nuclei are round and homogeneous. Some cells have small nucleoli (Papanicolaou, 16×).

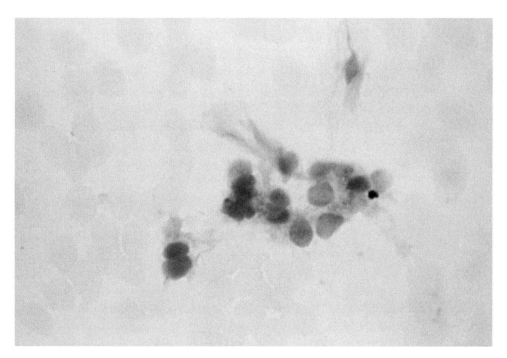

FIGURE 6-26. Serous cystadenoma. Small cluster of homogeneous cuboidal cells with numerous cytoplasmic, periodic acid–Schiff (PAS)-positive granules. The granules were digested with diastase (not shown) (PAS, 40×).

FIGURE 6-27. Serous cystadenoma. ThinPrep smear showing a small, monolayered cluster of cuboidal epithelium with finely vacuolated cytoplasm. The nuclei are round and uniform. The chromatin detail is lost (Papanicolaou, 63×).

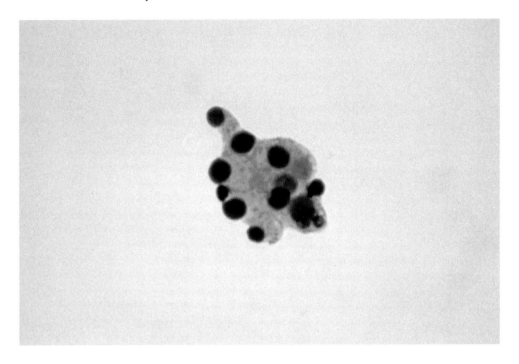

- Benign pancreatic ductal and acinar epithelium
- Mesothelial cells
- CPETs
- Endothelial neoplasms, such as hemangioma
- MCNs

Pancreatic ductal epithelium occurs in honeycombed sheets or groups. Large duct epithelium is columnar and contains cytoplasmic mucin, whereas the smaller ducts have scant, basophilic, dense, well-defined cytoplasm and apical mucin. Acinar cells occur in acinar-type aggregates or singly and are triangular, with abundant, dense, granular cytoplasm that contains PAS-positive, diastase-resistant zymogen granules and eccentric nuclei that have prominent nucleoli. Mesothelial cells are larger than SCA cells, are polygonal, and occur in flat sheets with windows.

CPET can be distinguished from serous cystadenoma by the salt-and-pepper chromatin pattern of the nuclei, wispy or dense cytoplasm, and demonstration of neuroendocrine differentiation by immunoperoxidase studies.

Hemangiomas produce elongated endothelial cells or sheets of smooth muscle.

MCN has a mucinous background and mucin-containing epithelium; the presence of either one of these excludes the diagnosis of SCA.

Mucinous Cystic Neoplasm and Mucinous Cystadenocarcinoma

MCN was the other cystic neoplasm defined by Compagno and Oertel in 1978 [68]. Compagno and Oertel recognized that all MCNs have the potential for malignant behavior,

regardless of the histopathologic features of the cells. The term *mucinous cystadenocarcinoma* is reserved for neoplasms showing invasion or distant metastases.

MCN and MCA occur chiefly in middle-aged women in the body or tail of the pancreas [68, 69]. Signs and symptoms are the result of a mass effect, but an increasing number are being discovered incidentally [3, 68]. The pancreatic ductal cell is believed to be the progenitor cell [70].

Grossly, most MCNs are multiloculated, with cysts of varying sizes filled with mucoid material, which imparts a gelatinous appearance to the cut surface (Figure 6-28). Unilocular variants also occur [3, 69]. Cystadenocarcinoma may show solid areas with necrosis. Microscopically, the cysts are lined by columnar, mucin-containing epithelium (Figure 6-29) that may form papillary projections or have nuclear atypia of varying degrees (Figure 6-30) [68, 69]. The cysts typically have an adjacent layer of dense stroma resembling ovarian stroma (see Figure 6-29) and an outer layer of hyalinized connective tissue [68, 69]. Flattened, nonmucinous epithelium may also be apparent [3, 69]. Under the World Health Organization classification, neoplasms with benign epithelium are referred to as *mucinous cystadenomas*, and neoplasms lined with dysplastic epithelium are referred to as *mucinous cystic tumor with moderate dysplasia*. The presence of even one mitotic figure in the lining epithelium has been associated with aggressive and malignant behavior [3]. Mucinous cystadenocarcinomas are lined by epithelium showing severe dysplasia/carcinoma in situ and frequent mitoses and may show stromal invasion or metastases (Figure 6-31) [71].

The fluid obtained by FNAB is usually clear to white and viscid. Cytologic preparations of MCN are

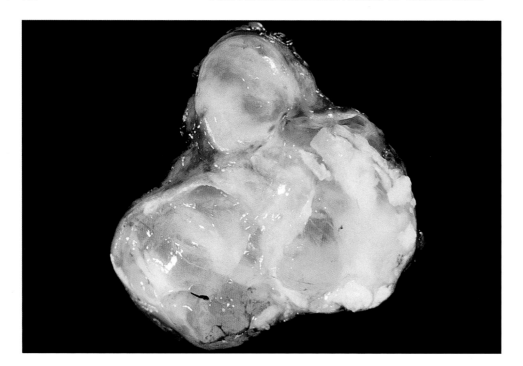

FIGURE 6-28. Mucinous cystic neoplasm. Gross appearance showing cut surface of multiloculated neoplasm containing numerous thin-walled cysts filled with gray-white mucoid material.

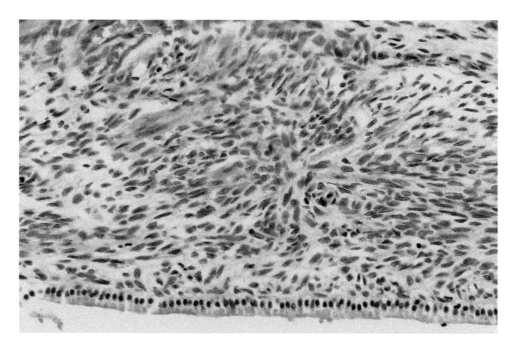

FIGURE 6-29. Mucinous cystic neoplasm. Resection specimen showing single layer of tall, columnar mucinous epithelium with an ovarian-type stroma. The nuclei are basally located and lack atypia (Hematoxylin and Eosin, 40×).

FIGURE 6-30. Mucinous cystic neoplasm. Resection specimen showing a pseudostratified epithelial lining that is thrown into papillary folds. The epithelium shows a loss of cytoplasmic mucin. The nuclei are hyperchromatic and more elongated (Hematoxylin and Eosin, 40×).

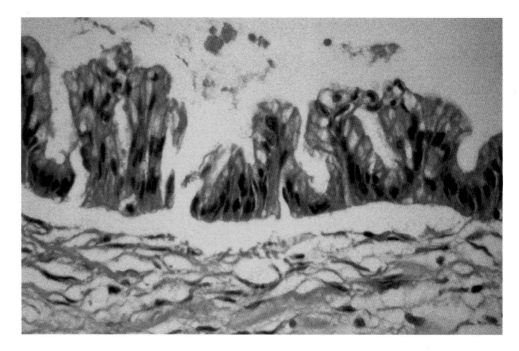

FIGURE 6-31. Mucinous cystadenocarcinoma. Resection specimen showing invasive, moderately differentiated adenocarcinoma, arising from a mucinous cystic neoplasm (*arrow*) (Hematoxylin and Eosin, 40×).

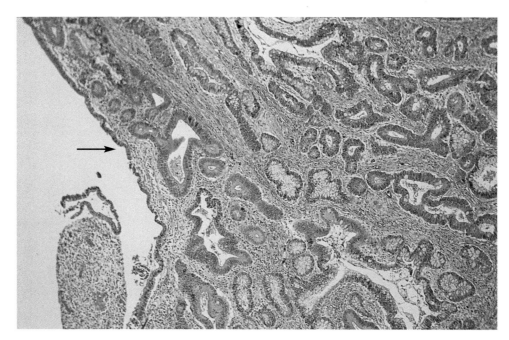

characterized by the presence of background mucin, evident even on ThinPrep smears. The cellularity varies from scant to moderate. The smears are composed of mucinous, columnar epithelium arranged in flat sheets (Figure 6-32) that may show pseudoacinar formations (Figure 6-33), papillary groups, palisading columns (Figure 6-34), or single cells. The cytoplasmic borders within the sheets are well defined (Figure 6-35). The nuclear atypia is minimal and characterized by slight elongation of the nuclei, nuclear membrane indentations and grooves, and a preserved nuclear-to-cytoplasmic ratio (Figure 6-36). The cytologic and architectural atypia varies in severity (Figure 6-37). Because the cyst lining is typically heterogeneous, malignancy cannot always be excluded. In some cases, the presence of background mucin and mucin-containing histiocytes are the only indicators of MCN. Special stains for mucin may increase the detection of mucin-containing epithelial cells or mucin within the

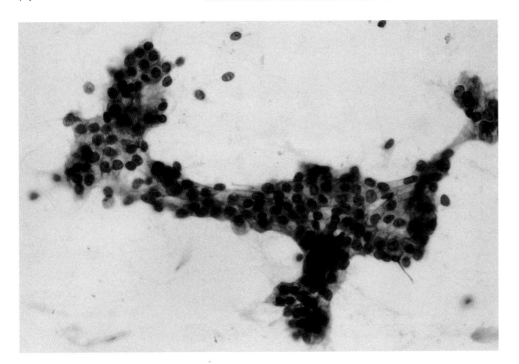

FIGURE 6-32. Mucinous cystic neoplasm. Flat, branching sheet of columnar mucinous epithelium. A few naked nuclei are present in the background (Papanicolaou, 25×).

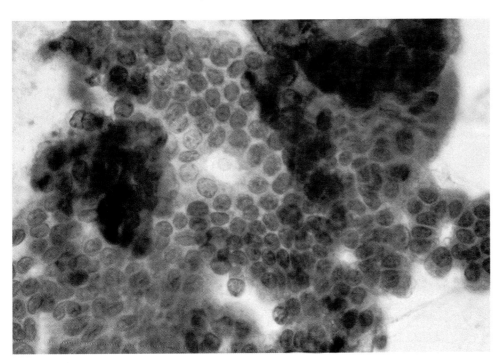

FIGURE 6-33. Mucinous cystic neoplasm. Flat sheet with pseudoacinar formations (Hematoxylin and Eosin, 40×).

FIGURE 6-34. Mucinous cystic neoplasm. Columnar mucinous epithelium in a palisaded, or picket fence, arrangement with background mucin (Hematoxylin and Eosin, 40×).

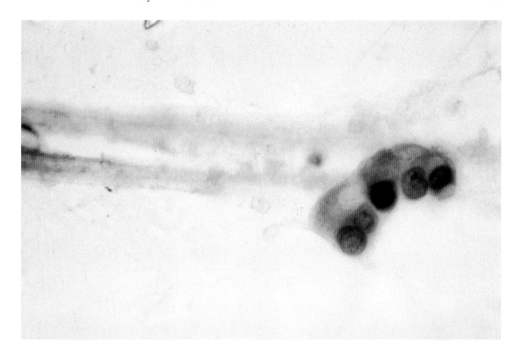

FIGURE 6-35. Mucinous cystic neoplasm. Flat sheet of columnar, mucinous epithelium showing sharp cytoplasmic borders. The cells have clear cytoplasm containing mucin (Papanicolaou, 40×).

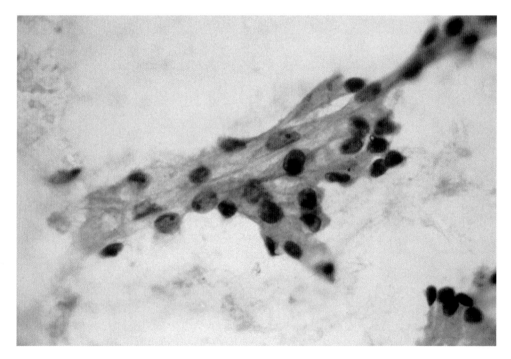

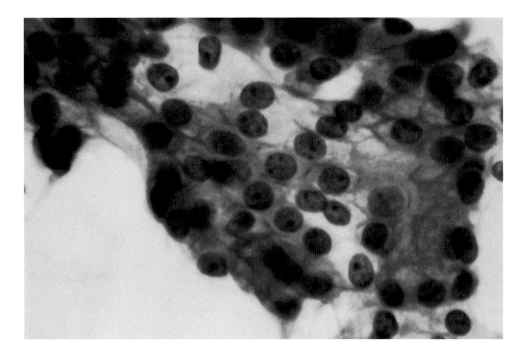

FIGURE 6-36. Mucinous cystic neoplasm. High-power view of Figure 6-32 showing round, relatively uniform nuclei with evenly distributed chromatin and small nucleoli (Papanicolaou, 40×).

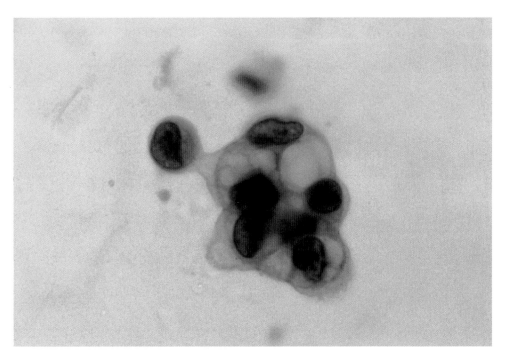

FIGURE 6-37. Mucinous cystic neoplasm. Papillary group showing an increased nuclear-to-cytoplasmic ratio, nuclear membrane irregularities, and irregular chromatin distribution. The atypia is insufficient for a diagnosis of malignancy in this neoplasm (Papanicolaou, 100×; ×1.6 optivar).

FIGURE 6-38. Mucinous cystic neoplasm. The smears were initially interpreted as consistent with a pseudocyst because of the granular background and inflammatory cells. A mucicarmine stain was ordered because of the presence of degenerated cells with a columnar shape seen on review (Papanicolaou, 40×).

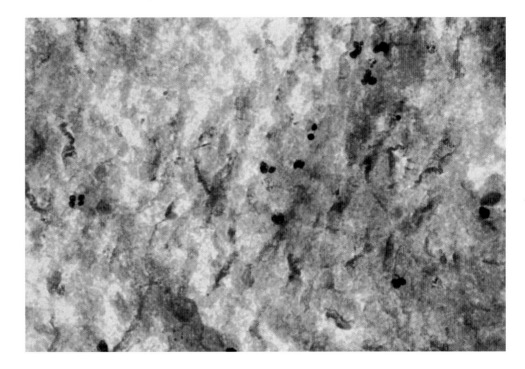

FIGURE 6-39. Mucinous cystic neoplasm. A mucicarmine stain performed on an additional slide of the case shown in Figure 6-37 shows background mucin and a single columnar cell with intracytoplasmic mucin (bottom). These findings are at least suggestive of a mucinous cystic neoplasm (Mucicarmine, 40×).

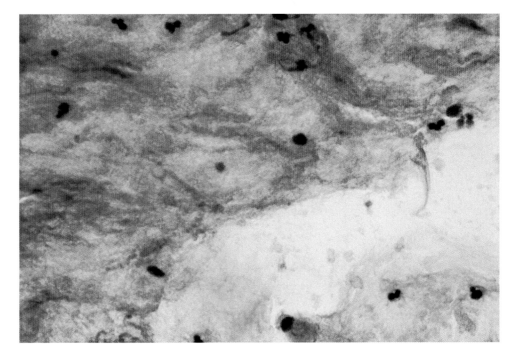

background and histiocytes (Figures 6-38 and 6-39). The additional slides prepared for mucin stains may contain epithelial cells not present on the original, Papanicolaou-stained smear (Figure 6-40).

Cytology of Mucinous Cystic Neoplasms

- Background mucin
- Columnar, mucinous epithelium
- Sheets, papillary groups, single cells, palisading groups
- Pseudoacinar formations
- Absence of cytomorphologic features of malignancy, necrosis, mitoses

MCAs may be invasive or noninvasive [71]. The radiologic correlate or MCA with invasion is a solid nodule seen within the wall of a pancreatic cystic lesion. Aspi-

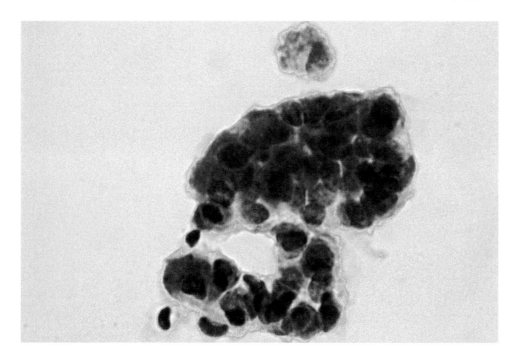

FIGURE 6-40. Mucinous cystic neoplasm. Papillary cluster of epithelial cells with a rim of cytoplasmic mucin. The Papanicolaou-stained smear lacked epithelial cells. This cluster was the only evidence for a mucinous cystic neoplasm in this case. The other cyst fluid markers had been misleading (alcian blue, 63×).

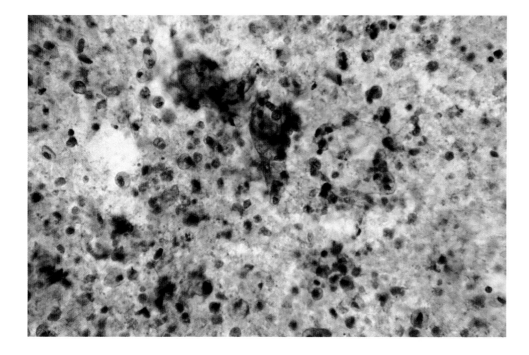

FIGURE 6-41. Mucinous cystadenocarcinoma. The smears are very cellular, and a dirty background with abundant necrosis is readily apparent (Papanicolaou, 20×).

ration of the solid mass will usually yield material diagnostic of malignancy, even when the cyst fluid does not. In contrast to MCNs, the cytologic sample from MCAs is typically very cellular, with blood and necrosis in the background (Figure 6-41). MCAs show more complex and varied architectural patterns. The cells may occur in flat sheets with exaggerated cell borders due to cytoplasmic mucin (Figure 6-42), in groups with acinar formations (Figure 6-43), and in papillary three-dimensional

groups (Figure 6-44). Cellular dyshesion is a prominent feature of MCAs; in some cases the cells may occur almost exclusively as single cells (Figure 6-45). Single cells with cytoplasmic vacuoles or signet-ring cells (Figure 6-46) may also be a prominent feature. The cells in MCAs show the cytomorphologic features of malignancy, such as increased nuclear-to-cytoplasmic ratio, nuclear membrane irregularities, and abnormalities of chromatin distribution (Figure 6-47). Individual cells or groups may

FIGURE 6-42. Mucinous cystadenocarcinoma. Loose aggregate of cells with an exaggerated honeycomb appearance due to abundant intracytoplasmic mucin. Numerous single cells are seen as well (Papanicolaou, 40×).

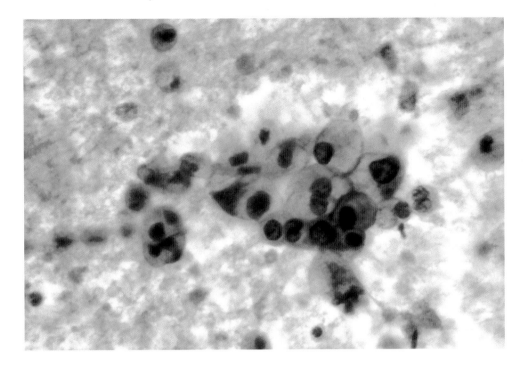

FIGURE 6-43. Mucinous cystadenocarcinoma. Group of malignant cells forming an acinus (Papanicolaou, 63×).

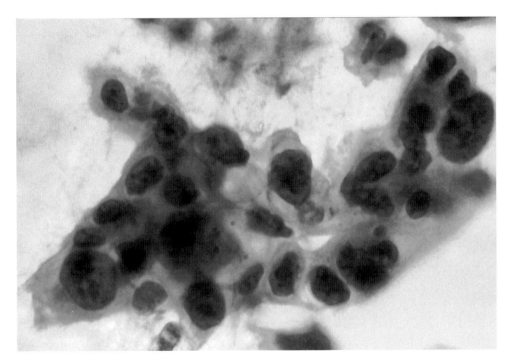

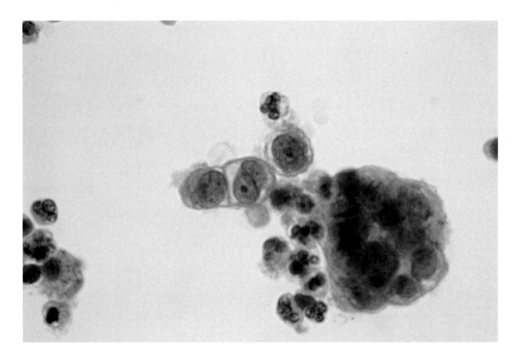

FIGURE 6-44. Mucinous cystadenocarcinoma. Papillary, three-dimensional cluster of malignant cells with single malignant cells (Papanicolaou, 63×).

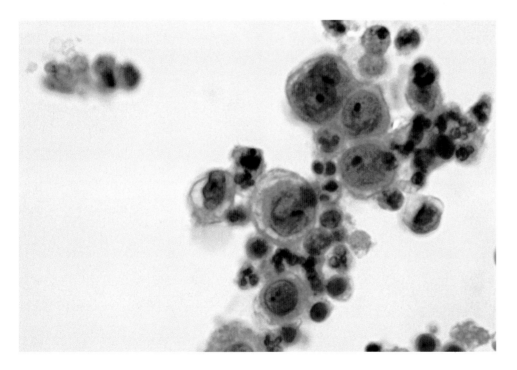

FIGURE 6-45. Mucinous cystadenocarcinoma. The malignant cells in this case occurred almost exclusively as single cells and were partially obscured by inflammation. The cells have a very high nuclear-to-cytoplasmic ratio, with irregular nuclear membranes that focally abut the cytoplasmic membrane. Nucleoli are prominent (Papanicolaou, 63×).

FIGURE 6-46. Mucinous cystadenocarcinoma. Signet-ring cells (Papanicolaou, 40×; ×1.6 optivar).

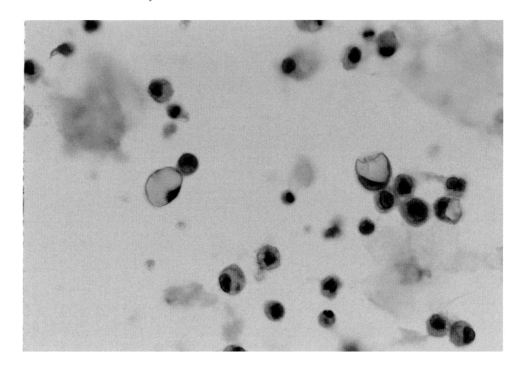

FIGURE 6-47. Mucinous cystadenocarcinoma. Flat sheet of malignant cells showing extreme anisonucleosis, nuclear membrane irregularities, and irregular chromatin clearing (Papanicolaou, 63×).

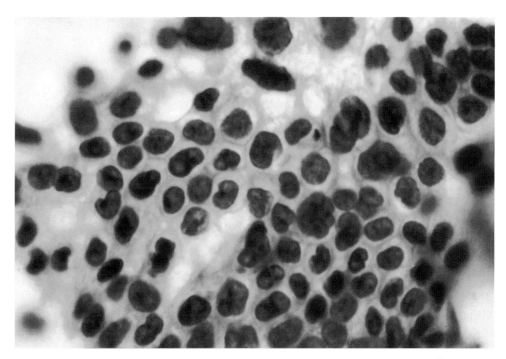

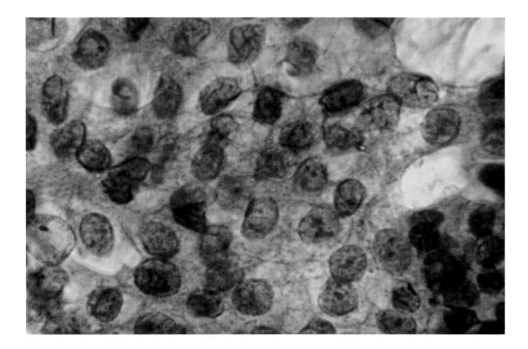

FIGURE 6-48. Mucinous cystadenocarcinoma. Flat, relatively cohesive sheet of well-differentiated adeno-carcinoma with subtle nuclear membrane alter-ations, irregularities in chromatin distribution, and hypochromasia (Papanico-laou, 63×).

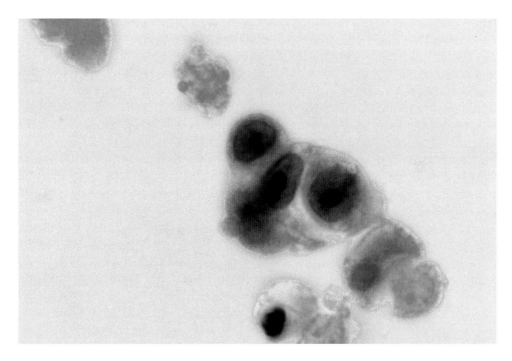

FIGURE 6-49. Mucinous cystadenocarcinoma. These malignant cells have promi-nent macronucleoli. Tumor ghost cells are seen in the background (Papanicolaou, 100×; ×1.6 optivar).

show more subtle features of malignancy (Figure 6-48) or lack features of malignancy. Some cases show promi-nent nucleoli (Figure 6-49). The presence of mitoses (Fig-ure 6-50) or coagulative necrosis (Figure 6-51), which produces tumor ghost cells, should raise the index of sus-picion for malignancy. A mucicarmine stain will demon-strate cytoplasmic mucin (Figure 6-52). Background mucin is a feature of MCAs as it is with MCNs. Cell

blocks show columnar epithelium with nuclear atypia, mitoses, and necrosis (Figure 6-53).

Cytology of Mucinous Cystadenocarcinoma

- Background mucin
- Mucinous epithelium with features of malignancy
- Sheets, papillary groups, single cells, signet-ring cells

FIGURE 6-50. Mucinous cystadenocarcinoma. The presence of mitoses, such as the one in this field, are associated with malignancy (Papanicolaou, 63×).

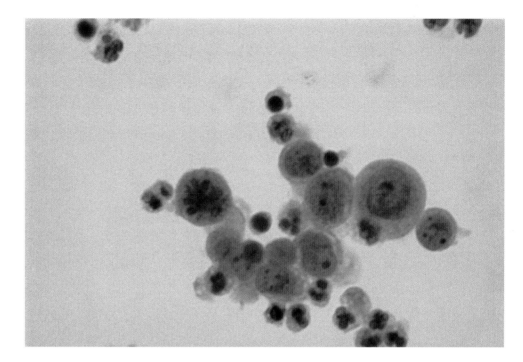

FIGURE 6-51. Mucinous cystadenocarcinoma. The cellularity in this specimen was relatively low, but there was abundant coagulative necrosis that produced tumor ghost cells, a feature of malignancy (Papanicolaou, 63×).

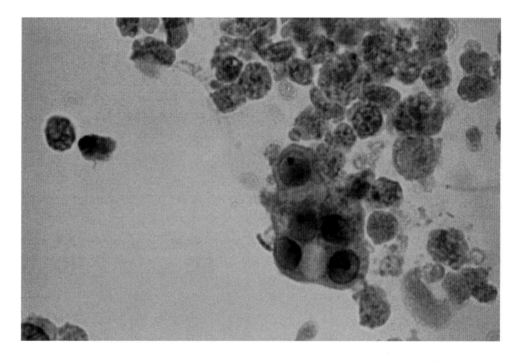

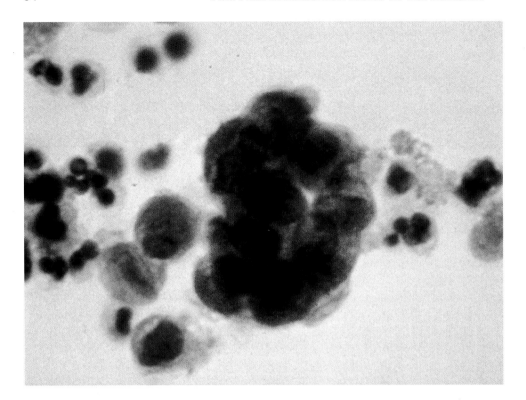

FIGURE 6-52. Mucinous cystadenocarcinoma. A mucicarmine stain performed on the case in Figure 6-43 demonstrates cytoplasmic mucin (mucicarmine, 40×).

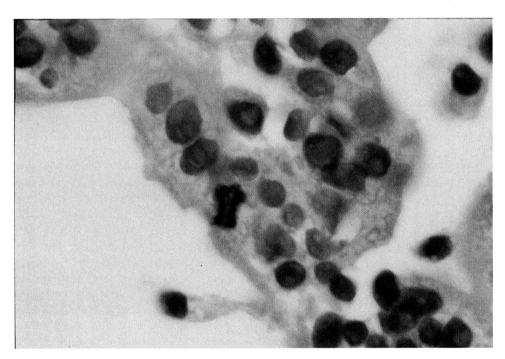

FIGURE 6-53. Mucinous cystadenocarcinoma. Cell block specimen showing columnar epithelium with nuclear atypia and a mitotic figure (Papanicolaou, 100×; ×1.6 optivar).

FIGURE 6-54. Intraductal papillary-mucinous tumor. Gross photograph shows a papillary neoplasm extending along the entire length of the pancreatic ductal system and dilating the pancreatic duct.

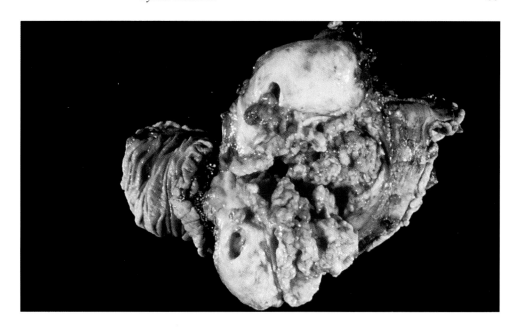

- Necrosis
- Mitoses
- Prominent nucleoli

The differential diagnosis includes the following (see also Table 6-2):

- Pseudocyst
- Retention cyst
- SCA
- SPPT
- Ductal carcinoma with cystic degeneration

As previously discussed, pseudocyst and SCA are excluded by the presence of mucin, whether it is in the background, in histiocytes, or in epithelial cells. Theoretically, retention cysts may produce a cyst that contains mucin because they communicate with the pancreatic duct. Fortunately, as previously stated, retention cysts are small and encountered relatively infrequently [1]. To date, all of the cysts containing mucin encountered in the MGH have been MCNs; however, aspirates from particularly small cysts that contain mucin and benign-appearing ductal-type mucinous epithelium should be regarded with some caution. Other cyst fluid markers will aid in the differential diagnosis. SPPT has a distinctive architectural pattern and lacks mucin within the neoplastic cells. Ductal carcinoma with mucinous differentiation may not be readily distinguished from MCA, but this distinction is not necessary.

Intraductal Papillary-Mucinous Tumors

Intraductal or invasive papillary-mucinous carcinoma and intraductal papillary mucinous tumor (World Health Orga-

nization classification) [71] are recently defined entities with a clinicopathologic presentation distinct from that of MCN and MCA [72]. They have previously been referred to as *intraductal mucinous hypersecreting neoplasms*, *mucinous ductal ectasia*, *ductectatic mucinous cystadenoma* or *cystadenocarcinoma*, *intraductal papillary neoplasms*, and *papillary cystadenomas* or *cystadenocarcinoma* [72, 73]. These neoplasms occur primarily in elderly patients, show a male predilection [72], occur in the head and body [74], and present with symptoms that mimic chronic or relapsing pancreatitis [72, 73]. The ERCP and duodenal endoscopic findings are pathognomonic, showing extreme dilation of the entire length of the main pancreatic duct, with side branch ectasia in the absence of a pancreatic duct stricture [72] and a dilated ampulla through which is secreted abundant, viscid mucus [75]. CT or transabdominal ultrasound findings may be the initial studies performed, and they may show only pancreatic cysts, thereby entering intraductal papillary-mucinous tumor into the differential diagnosis of pancreatic cystic lesions.

Macroscopically, specimens typically show no mass lesions unless there is a large invasive component. The main pancreatic duct is dilated and contains a papillary, complex proliferation (Figure 6-54). On histomorphology, the normal duct epithelium is replaced by mucin-producing columnar epithelium, with some goblet cells and varying amounts of papillary growth (Figures 6-55 and 6-56) and of cytologic atypia. The adjacent pancreatic parenchyma typically shows chronic pancreatitis.

Experience with the preoperative cytologic diagnoses of these neoplasms is limited. Tissue specimens, including aspiration cytology, brush cytology, and pancreatic biopsy, have been reported to have a high false-negative rate and to be helpful only when positive [72].

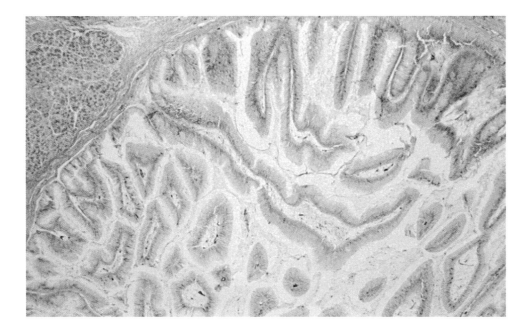

Figure 6-55. Intraductal papillary-mucinous tumor. Cross section of pancreatic duct from a resection specimen showing intraluminal papillary proliferation of neoplastic cells with scant mucin production. Nuclear atypia is minimal (Hematoxylin and Eosin, 10×).

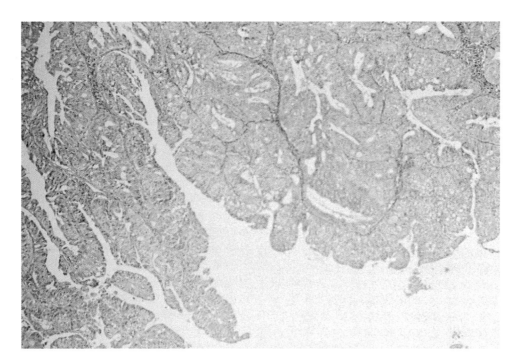

Figure 6-56. Intraductal papillary-mucinous carcinoma. Luminal surface of pancreatic duct from resection specimen showing a papillary neoplasm with a complex architecture, including cribriform spaces (Hematoxylin and Eosin, 20×).

One prospective study of 14 patients, however, showed a sensitivity, specificity, and overall accuracy of 91%, 100%, and 93% for cytologic examination of pancreatic secretions [76].

The cytologic findings are as varied as the histopathologic findings and overlap with those of MCN and MCA. Cytologic preparations from benign lesions show mucinous epithelium in honeycombed sheets with well-defined cytoplasmic borders and minimal cytologic atypia (Figure 6-57)

with background mucin. The cytology of lesions of intermediate malignant potential has not been described, but the cytologic findings probably parallel those seen in histopathology and would be characterized by increasing architectural complexity and cytologic atypia. The intraductal papillary-mucinous carcinomas produce cellular smears composed of cells with the cytomorphologic features of malignancy in papillary groups (Figure 6-58), small loose groups, or singly. The presence of necrosis is

FIGURE 6-57. Intraductal papillary-mucinous tumor. Sheet of columnar mucinous epithelium. Such epithelium may be seen to originate either from a mucinous cystic neoplasm or an intraductal papillary-mucinous tumor (Papanicolaou, 40×). (Courtesy of Dr. William J. Frable, Virginia Commonwealth University/Medical College of Virginia School of Medicine, Richmond, VA.)

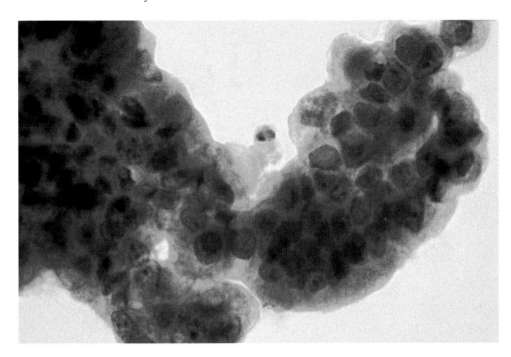

FIGURE 6-58. Invasive papillary-mucinous carcinoma. Three-dimensional papillary group with a smooth border. The nuclei are crowded together, are pleomorphic, and have prominent nucleoli (Papanicolaou, 40×).

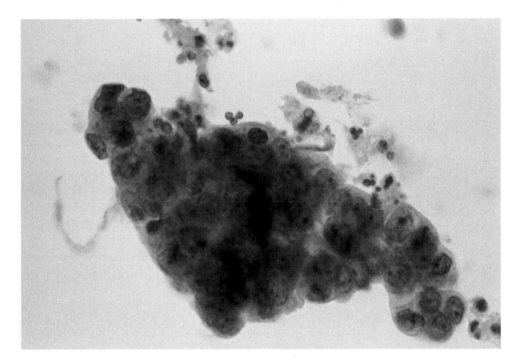

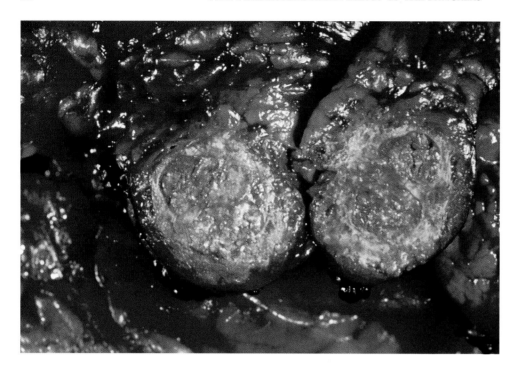

FIGURE 6-59. Solid pseudopapillary tumor. Gross photograph showing well-circumscribed, tan tumor in the pancreas with yellow areas of necrosis.

suggestive of invasion, but the distinction between an intraductal papillary-mucinous carcinoma and an invasive one may not be reliable on cytology alone.

Cytology of Intraductal Papillary-Mucinous Tumors

- Variable cellularity
- Papillary groups
- Variable cytologic atypia, depending on degree of differentiation
- Variable mucinous differentiation

The cytologic differential diagnosis is similar to that of MCN and MCA (see Table 6-2).

Solid Pseudopapillary Tumor

This entity has also been referred to as papillary-cystic neoplasm, solid and cystic tumor of the pancreas, papillary cystic tumor of the pancreas, and papillary epithelial neoplasm of the pancreas. *SPPT* is the term proposed under the World Health Organization classification [71]. SPPT is an uncommon neoplasm of low malignant potential occurring primarily in young women (mean age of 24 years) [77, 78] and presenting as a large, asymptomatic abdominal mass. These neoplasms have a good prognosis and are usually cured by complete surgical resection [78–80]. Metastases to the liver and extensive local invasion have been reported [78, 81, 82], but even patients with metastatic disease may have a good prognosis [81, 82].

Immunohistochemical and electron microscopic studies show evidence of differentiation of all the components of the pancreas, suggesting development from primitive pancreatic epithelial cells [83].

Grossly, the tumors are typically well encapsulated, composed of white-tan tissue, and have cystic and solid spaces with areas of hemorrhage and necrosis (Figure 6-59). Microscopically, the tumors are very cellular, with solid areas and cystic areas of hemorrhage and degeneration that may contain cholesterol crystals (Figure 6-60). The solid areas are composed of small, uniform tumor cells that surround fibrovascular cores with a layer of myxoid-mucinous stroma (Figure 6-61). PAS or alcian blue stains demonstrate the mucinous stroma of the fibrovascular cores (Figure 6-62).

Various authors have described the cytologic findings [84–87]. The smears are typically highly cellular and contain numerous straight or branching papillary structures (Figure 6-63). At the center is a delicate fibrovascular core (Figure 6-64) surrounded by a layer of myxoid stroma, which is lined by a variably thick layer of monomorphic neoplastic cells with round to oval nuclei having finely dispersed chromatin, small nucleoli (Figure 6-65) and occasional nuclear grooves or inclusions (Figure 6-66). The cytoplasm is amphophilic and occasionally contains PAS-positive granules. The hallmark is balls of myxoid or mucinous stromal material that may or may not be rimmed by a layer of neoplastic cells (Figure 6-67).

Cytology of Solid Pseudopapillary Tumor

- Very cellular
- Hallmark is balls or globules of myxoid stroma ± rim of neoplastic cells

FIGURE 6-60. Solid pseudopapillary tumor. Histologically, these tumors are characterized by cystic, solid, and pseudopapillary areas. The cystic areas are blood-filled in this case, and the pseudopapillary areas contain fibrovascular cores (Hematoxylin and Eosin, 10×).

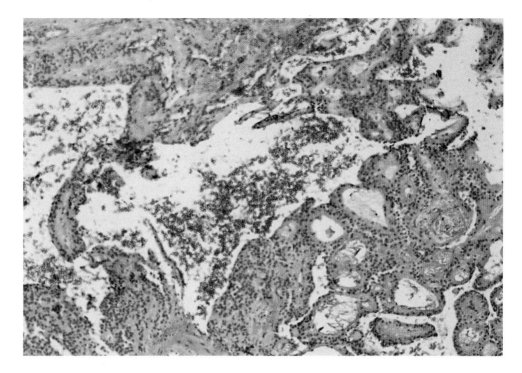

FIGURE 6-61. Solid pseudopapillary tumor. Homogeneous population of neoplastic cells with round to oval nuclei containing small nucleoli and having scant cytoplasm surrounding a fibrovascular core with a myxoid stroma (Hematoxylin and Eosin, 40×).

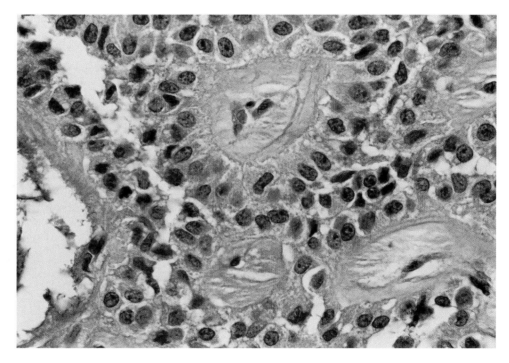

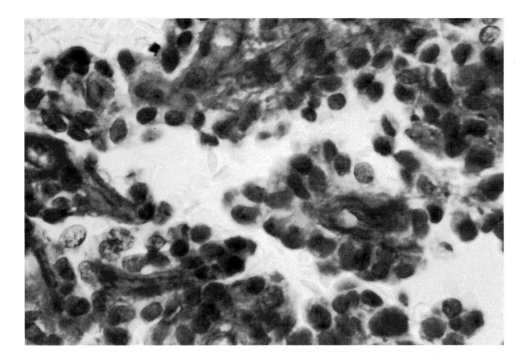

FIGURE 6-62. Solid pseudopapillary tumor. Cell block specimen showing numerous papillary fragments. A periodic acid–Schiff (PAS) stain demonstrates the mucin within the myxoid stroma (PAS, 40×). (Case courtesy of Dr. Edmund S. Cibas, Brigham and Women's Hospital, Harvard Medical School, Boston.)

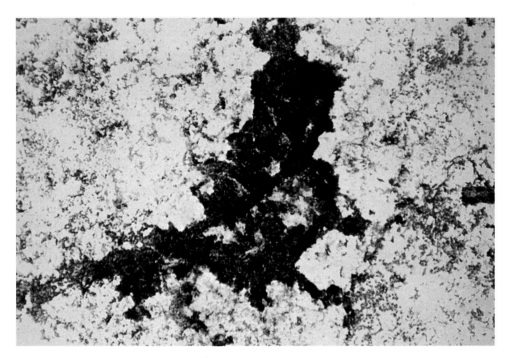

FIGURE 6-63. Solid pseudopapillary tumor. Fine needle aspiration biopsy smears are typically very cellular and contain numerous, branching fragments of tissue (Papanicolaou, 10×). (Case courtesy of Dr. Edmund S. Cibas, Brigham and Women's Hospital, Harvard Medical School, Boston.)

FIGURE 6-64. Solid pseudopapillary tumor. The neoplastic cells surround a central, fibrovascular core (Papanicolaou, 20×). (Case courtesy of Dr. Edmund S. Cibas, Brigham and Women's Hospital, Harvard Medical School, Boston.)

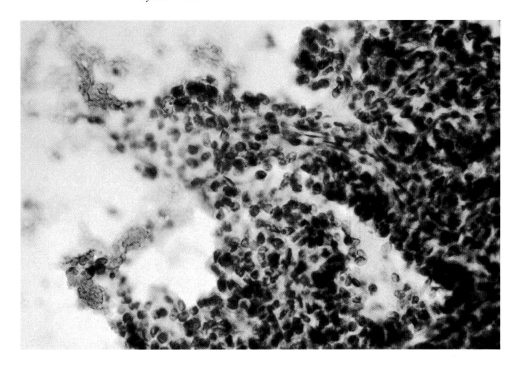

FIGURE 6-65. Solid pseudopapillary tumor. The nuclei are centrally placed, round to oval, with bland chromatin and micronucleoli. The cytoplasm is scant, wispy, and basophilic (Papanicolaou, 40×). (Case courtesy of Dr. Edmund S. Cibas, Brigham and Women's Hospital, Harvard Medical School, Boston.)

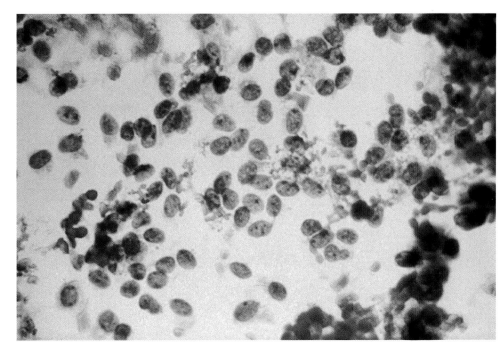

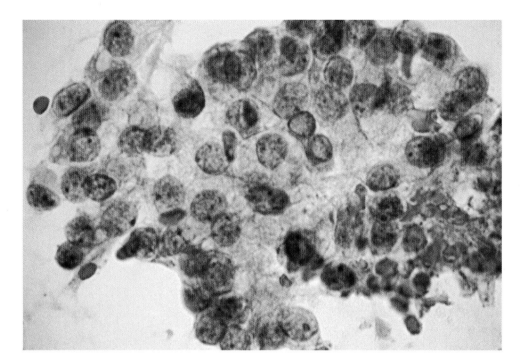

FIGURE 6-66. Solid pseudopapillary tumor. The nuclei may occasionally have intranuclear inclusions and nuclear grooves (Papanicolaou, 63×). (Case courtesy of Dr. Edmund S. Cibas, Brigham and Women's Hospital, Harvard Medical School, Boston.)

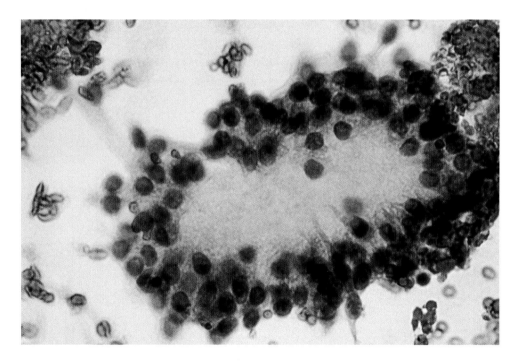

FIGURE 6-67. Solid pseudopapillary tumor. Neoplastic cells surrounding a myxoid stromal ball. This is a pathognomonic finding (Papanicolaou, 40×). (Case courtesy of Dr. Edmund S. Cibas, Brigham and Women's Hospital, Harvard Medical School, Boston.)

FIGURE 6-68. Cystic pancreatic endocrine tumor. Gross photograph showing well-defined, encapsulated cystic mass with residual tan-white tissue at the periphery of the cyst cavity.

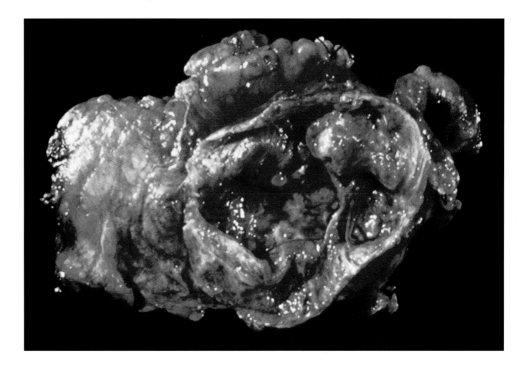

• Straight or branching papillary structures with delicate fibrovascular core with myxoid stroma
• Monomorphic epithelial cells with round to oval nuclei, finely dispersed chromatin, nuclear indentation or grooves, and small nucleoli
• Scant and ill-defined, vacuolated amphophilic cytoplasm, occasionally with PAS-positive granules or vacuolization
• Necrosis and macrophages in background

The differential diagnosis includes the following (see also Table 6-2):

• MCN
• CPET
• Acinar cell carcinoma
• Adenocarcinoma

MCN is characterized by mucinous epithelium of various grades of differentiation in a mucinous background, both features lacking in SPPT. Furthermore, MCN lacks the pathognomic feature of SPPT.

CPET produces aspirate smears composed of a homogeneous cell population, but the nuclei have a salt-and-pepper chromatin pattern, and the architectural features of SPPT are lacking.

Acinar cell carcinomas may be readily differentiated from SPPT by their abundant, well-defined cytoplasm that contains zymogen granules and by their large central to eccentric nuclei with prominent nucleoli.

Adenocarcinomas exhibit all the features of malignancy unequivocally lacking in SPPT.

Cystic Pancreatic Endocrine Tumors (Islet Cell Tumors)

Traditionally, CPET has been regarded as rare, representing 4.3% of all pancreatic endocrine tumors and 5.4% of all cystic neoplasms. One study, however, showed that cystic degeneration was relatively common among nonhyperfunctioning, large (8.4 cm in mean diameter) pancreatic endocrine tumors [88]. One reason for the discrepancy may be that earlier reports focused on tumors that were predominantly cystic [88]. Because the majority of CPETs are nonfunctional, preoperative diagnosis presents a problem [88–90]. Nonfunctioning tumors may be confused preoperatively with pseudocyst or other pancreatic cystic neoplasms. One study suggested that the larger size of the tumor correlated with calcification and malignant behavior [88].

The most common location is in the body or tail. The cysts may be unilocular or multilocular, are lined by tan-white tissue (Figure 6-68), and may contain blood. Histologically, they resemble their solid counterparts (Figure 6-69). Although the exact histogenesis of CPET is not known, it is thought to develop as a result of ischemia with infarction or possibly from hemorrhage within an endocrine tumor [91, 92].

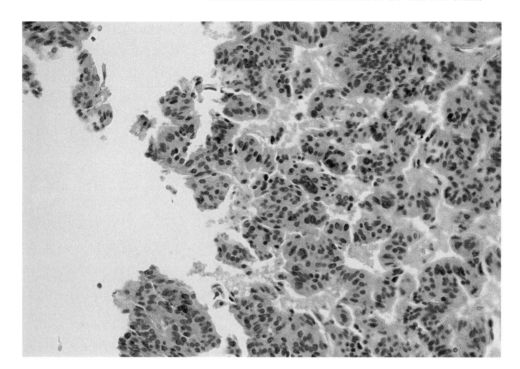

FIGURE 6-69. Cystic pancreatic endocrine tumor. Nest of homogeneous tumor cells with uniform nuclei having a salt-and-pepper chromatin pattern (Hematoxylin and Eosin, 40×).

FNAB slide preparations are moderately cellular (Figure 6-70). The cells are homogeneous, generally occurring in small aggregates, clusters, or singly. The oval to round nuclei may be centrally placed or eccentric, imparting a plasmacytoid appearance. The nuclear membranes are smooth, and the chromatin is finely granular and evenly dispersed. Small nucleoli may be seen (Figures 6-71 to 6-73). The cytoplasm is basophilic and may be wispy or dense and well defined. Abundant blood may be present in the background. Immunocytochemical and electron microscopic studies reveal neuroendocrine differentiation (Figure 6-74). Rare reports have described the results of cyst fluid analysis. Low levels of CEA and CA 125, low viscosity, and variable amylase levels have been reported. One functioning tumor had elevated hormone levels in the cyst fluid [89].

Cytology of Cystic Pancreatic Endocrine Tumors

- Homogeneous cell population
- Clusters or single cells
- Monomorphic nuclei with salt-and-pepper chromatin, small nucleoli
- Basophilic cytoplasm, wispy or well defined
- Blood in the background
- Occasional plasmacytoid appearance

The cytologic differential diagnosis includes the following (see also Table 6-2):

- Mesothelial cells
- SCA
- SPPT
- Other neoplasms

Mesothelial cells occur in flat sheets with windows and lack both the salt-and-pepper chromatin pattern typical of CPETs as well as evidence of neuroendocrine differentiation. The differential diagnosis with SCA and SPPT have been previously discussed. The differential diagnosis of CPET is similar to its noncystic counterpart, which is discussed in Chapter 7.

Acinar Cell Cystadenocarcinoma

This neoplasm is exceedingly rare. Only three cases have been reported to date [93, 95]. Grossly they resemble SCA. The cyst-lining cells have the morphologic features of acinar cells of the pancreas. To date, no reports have described the cytomorphologic findings of acinar cell cystadenocarcinoma, although correct preoperative diagnosis using a CT-guided needle aspiration of one case has been reported [95].

A solid acinar cell carcinoma may undergo cystic degeneration and present as a cystic mass.

Vascular Tumors

Hemangiomas and lymphangiomas are included in the differential diagnosis of pancreatic cystic lesions, although both of these entities are rare in the pancreas. Only eight cases of pancreatic hemangioma have been reported in the literature [96]. Radiologic studies of hemangiomas are reportedly diagnostic [96]. Approximately 33 cases of lymphangioma of the pancreas have been reported [97–100]. They occur more frequently in women and in the body

FIGURE 6-70. Cystic pancreatic endocrine tumor. Fine needle aspiration biopsy smears of this specimen are very cellular. The neoplastic cells are arranged in loose clusters and singly. Abundant blood is seen in the background (Papanicolaou, 40×).

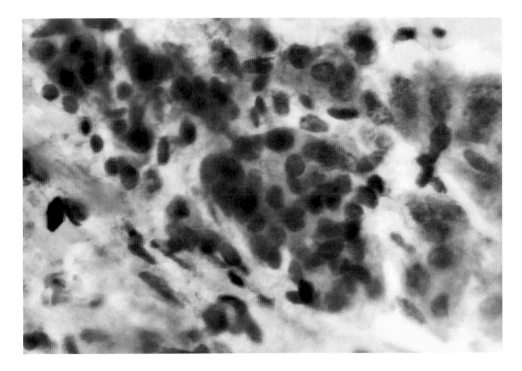

FIGURE 6-71. Cystic pancreatic endocrine tumor. The neoplastic cells are arranged in a flat sheet. The nuclei are homogeneous (Papanicolaou, 40×).

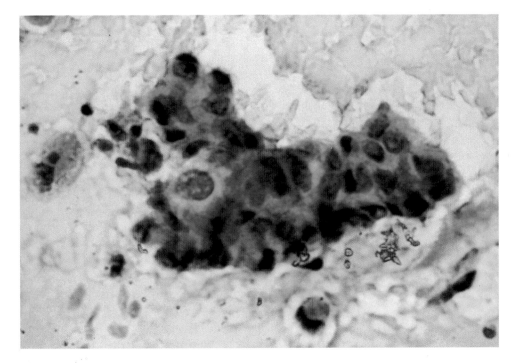

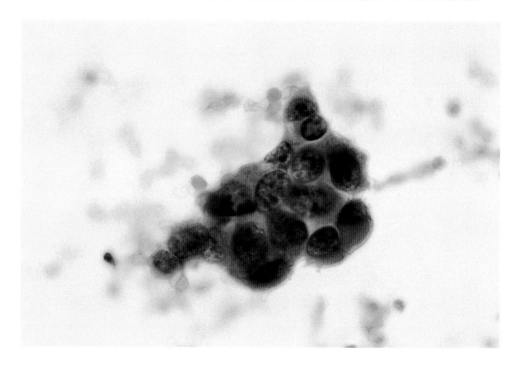

FIGURE 6-72. Cystic pancreatic endocrine tumor. Tight cluster of neoplastic cells with round, central to eccentric nuclei with coarsely stippled chromatin. The cytoplasm is dense and basophilic. Although the nuclei appear hyperchromatic, the nuclear membranes are smooth and regular, and the cells lack macronucleoli, distinguishing them from adenocarcinoma (Papanicolaou, 100×; ×1.6 optivar).

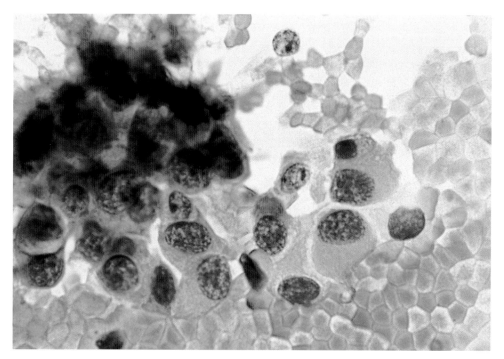

FIGURE 6-73. Cystic pancreatic endocrine tumor. Neoplastic cells with a plasmacytoid appearance (Papanicolaou, 100×).

FIGURE 6-74. Cystic pancreatic endocrine tumor. A chromogranin stain demonstrates cytoplasmic staining (immunoperoxidase, chromogranin, 40×).

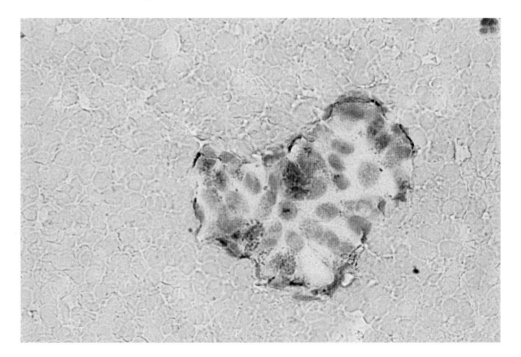

and tail of the pancreas than in the head [97]. On CT scan, they resemble SCA [97]. Histologically, they are also difficult to distinguish from SCA, but lymphangiomas are lined by flattened endothelial cells that lack glycogen and the cystic spaces are filled with lymph fluid [97]. The gross and histopathologic findings of both entities are similar to those of the tumor found in other locations.

The FNAB of one reported case of pancreatic hemangioma obtained 15–20 ml of sanguineous fluid that produced a nondiagnostic specimen [101]. FNAB of a pancreatic hemangioma seen in our department obtained copious amounts of blood. Smooth muscle with elongated, uniform nuclei in sheets without evidence of cytoplasmic borders were obtained (Figure 6-75). The endothelial cells occurred singly. The nuclei in some of the single cells were rounder, with indentations or minimal irregularities (Figure 6-76). Some cells had elongated, slightly vacuolated cytoplasm (Figure 6-77).

One report of an FNAB of a pancreatic lymphangioma described nondiagnostic acellular debris [100]. The aspirates of lymphangioma from other sites typically produce clear fluid and are scantly cellular. The cell population is typically composed of lymphocytes, a few histiocytes, and few endothelial cells.

Cytology of Benign Vascular Tumors

- Scant endothelial cells, singly or in sheets
- ± Smooth muscle from vessel walls
- ± Blood
- ± Other inflammatory cells

The differential diagnosis, discussed in the section on SCA, includes other cystic neoplasms, particularly SCA.

PERIPANCREATIC OR RETROPERITONEAL CYSTS OR NEOPLASMS

Peripancreatic or retroperitoneal processes, cysts, or neoplasms with cystic degeneration comprise a significant percentage of entities diagnosed radiologically as pancreatic cysts, accounting for 21% of cases in a prospective series of 28 cases [14]. In the series by Sperti et al. [95], they constituted only 4.7% of the total number of cases, but their series was much larger. Individual case reports also exist [102]. Reported entities are listed in Table 6-3. The possibility of a peripancreatic or retroperitoneal process should always be considered in the differential diagnosis of a pancreatic cyst.

Peritoneal Inclusion Cyst

Peritoneal inclusion cysts may present as an abdominal cyst, possibly pancreatic in origin [14]. The fluid is yellow and cloudy. ThinPrep smears show numerous single cells with abundant, basophilic cytoplasm demonstrating degenerative vacuolization in some cells and a fuzzy border on others. The nuclei are round to oval and eccentrically placed. These cells may be associated with a mixed inflammatory cell infiltrate composed of histio-

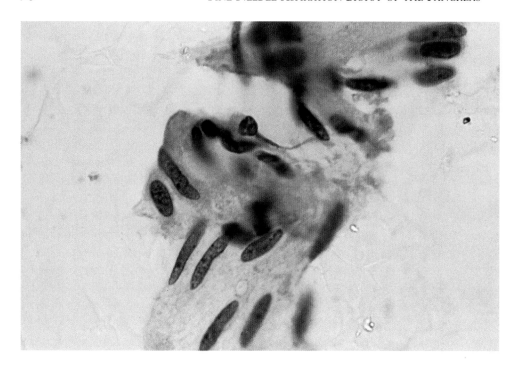

FIGURE 6-75. Hemangioma. The smooth muscle cells have elongated, bland, uniform nuclei. The cytoplasm is relatively abundant, but the cytoplasmic borders are indistinct (Hematoxylin and Eosin, 100×).

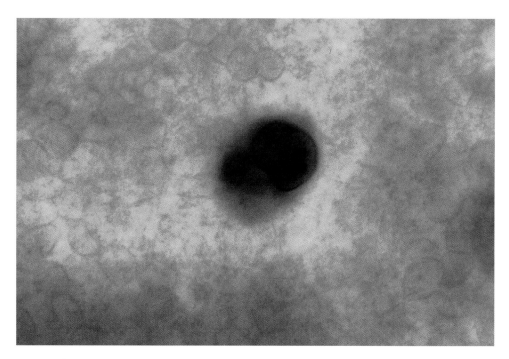

FIGURE 6-76. Hemangioma. Occasional cells may be rounded with minimal nuclear indentation (Hematoxylin and Eosin, 100×; ×1.6 optivar).

FIGURE 6-77. Hemangioma. Other single cells were elongated with slight irregularities in nuclear shape (Hematoxylin and Eosin, 100×).

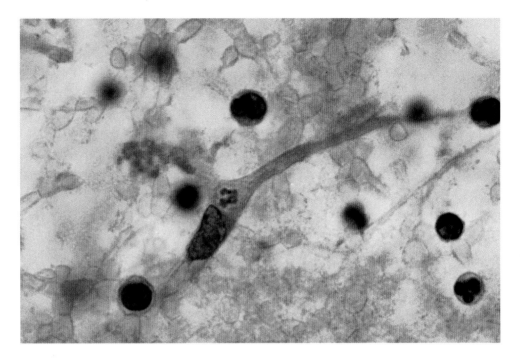

TABLE 6-3. Nonpancreatic Cysts Presenting as Pancreatic Cysts

Location	Number of Cases
Gastrointestinal stromal tumor arising from gastric wall	1
Gastrointestinal papillary carcinoma	1
Mesothelial inclusion cyst	2
Retroperitoneal serous cystadenoma	1
Adrenal cyst	4
Retroperitoneal leiomyoma with cystic degeneration	1
Lymphoma with cystic degeneration	1
Mesenteric cyst	1
Left hydronephrosis	1
Mesenteric lymphangioma	1
Gastric epithelioid leiomyosarcoma	1

Sources: Data from BA Centeno, AL Warshaw, W Mayo-Smith, et al. Cytological diagnosis of pancreatic cystic lesions: a prospective study of 28 percutaneous aspirates. Acta Cytol 1997;41:972; C Sperti, F Cappellazzo, C Pasquali, et al. Cystic neoplasms of the pancreas: problems in differential diagnosis. Am Surg 1993;59:740; and R Malhotra, R Evans, J Bhawan, et al. A malignant gastric leiomyoblastoma presenting as an infected pseudocyst of the pancreas. Am J Gastroenterol 1988;83:452.

FIGURE 6-78. Peritoneal inclusion cyst. Mesothelial cell with histiocytes (Papanicolaou, 40×; ×1.6 optivar).

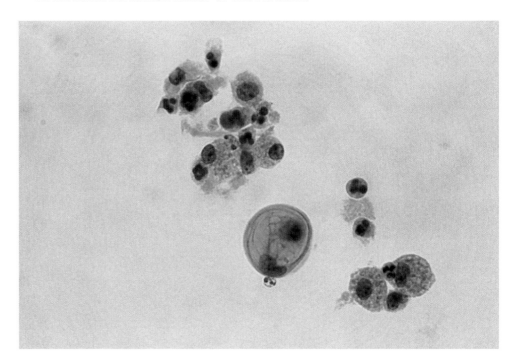

FIGURE 6-79. Peritoneal inclusion cyst. Large mesothelial cell with cytoplasmic vacuolization (Papanicolaou, 20×).

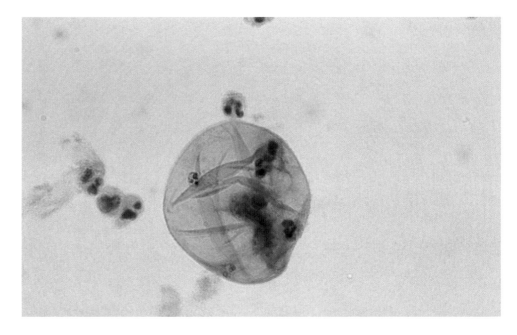

cytes, lymphocytes, and rare neutrophils (Figures 6-78 and 6-79).

Cytology of Peritoneal Inclusion Cyst

- Round cells
- Basophilic cytoplasmic with fuzzy borders or degenerative changes
- Eccentric nuclei with no atypia

If the site of origin is not known, definitive diagnosis may not be possible. The differential diagnosis includes other benign entities:

- Simple cyst
- Serous cystadenoma

The mesothelial cells are typically larger than the cells of these entities. This feature, along with precise clinical information, may aid diagnosis.

Gastrointestinal Stromal Tumor

The following provides a description of a gastrointestinal stromal tumor taken from this author's experience. The cell block from a gastrointestinal stromal tumor (GIST)

FIGURE 6-80. Gastrointestinal stromal tumor. Low-power view of cell block showing stromal fragment and blood (Hematoxylin and Eosin, 10×; ×1.25 optivar).

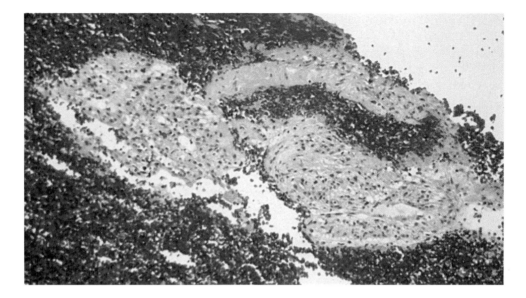

FIGURE 6-81. Gastrointestinal stromal tumor. High-power view showing spindle cells with minimal nuclear atypia and no necrosis or mitoses (Hematoxylin and Eosin, 40×; ×1.6 optivar).

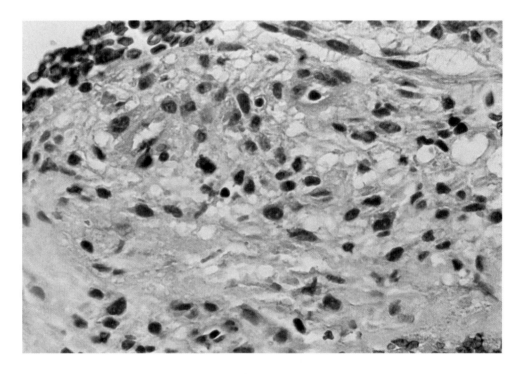

aspirated under the radiologic impression that it originated from the pancreas was sent to this author in consultation because the radiologic impression had confounded interpretation of the FNAB findings: The referring pathologist did not consider the possibility of a GIST because of the erroneous clinical information of a "pancreatic cystic lesion." The cell block specimen showed tissue fragments composed of homogeneous, spindle cells with scant eosinophilic cytoplasm (Figure

6-80). The stroma was loose in some areas. No mitoses, nuclear atypia, or necrosis were seen (Figure 6-81).

Cytology of Gastrointestinal Stromal Tumor

- Cellular fragments
- Spindle cells
- Myxoid, loose, or dense stroma
- Necrosis, mitoses, and nuclear atypia may be variably present

The differential diagnosis includes other mesenchymal neoplasms with cystic degeneration, but the cytomorphology characterized by the presence of spindle cells excludes pancreatic epithelial neoplasms such as SCA and MCN.

ACCURACY AND USEFULNESS OF PANCREATIC CYST FLUID CYTOLOGY

In a retrospective series of 31 and a prospective series of 28 FNABs of pancreatic cysts from MGH, the sensitivity of cytology alone for the detection of carcinoma was 71% for the retrospective and 67% for the prospective series [13, 14]. These reported studies, as well as our ongoing experience with these entities, have shown that cytology alone, with the addition of special stains for mucin, can distinguish mucinous from nonmucinous lesions in most cases and correctly diagnose rare entities when an adequately cellular sample is obtained. No false-positive diagnoses have been made to date at MGH.

The most common diagnostic pitfalls in the cytologic interpretation of cystic neoplasms include the following:

1. Nonrepresentative samples from cystic neoplasms
2. Obscuring inflammation, necrosis, or debris
3. Innocuous-appearing neoplastic epithelium
4. Gastrointestinal epithelium
5. Peripancreatic or retroperitoneal cysts appearing as pancreatic in origin on imaging studies

The cyst fluids from cystic neoplasms sometimes lack diagnostic cells. This occurs frequently with SCA but is a problem with other cystic neoplasms as well. Some MCNs may have only mucin-containing histiocytes and background mucin in their aspirates, or the epithelial cells may be degenerated and not readily seen. Special stains for mucin, such as mucicarmine and alcian blue, demonstrate the background mucin, mucin-containing histiocytes, and degenerated mucinous epithelium. A further benefit of performing cytochemical stains for mucin is that the additional slides prepared for mucin stains may contain epithelial cells not present on the original slides, whose presence is further highlighted by the mucin stains. Mucinous cystadenocarcinomas may also produce cyst fluids that lack diagnostic cells. Mucin stains performed on additional slides will identify the cyst fluid as originating in a mucinous neoplasm, as for MCNs. In most cases, however, malignant neoplasms have solid areas associated with the cyst. In such cases, aspiration of the solid area usually yields diagnostic material [103]. Some samples will lack any neoplastic epithelium or mucin. In such cases, differentiation from pseudocyst may not be possible.

Because cystic neoplasms may be accompanied by inflammation and degeneration that may obscure the neoplastic cells, they may be underdiagnosed. Cyst aspirates should be approached with a high index of suspicion for cystic neoplasms, particularly mucinous neoplasms. Mucin stains will help identify obscured mucinous epithelium.

Unlike the first pitfall, in the third pitfall, neoplastic epithelium may be present but may not be recognized as such because it is bland or benign in appearance and leads to a diagnosis of pseudocyst. The presence of any epithelium in a pancreatic cyst aspirate, unless it is normal pancreatic epithelium or a contaminant, excludes the diagnosis of pseudocyst.

Normal gastrointestinal epithelium, obtained most frequently when FNAB is performed under endoscopic ultrasonography (EUS) guidance, presents a diagnostic dilemma because the diagnosis of MCN rests on the identification of mucinous epithelium. The background mucin associated with normal gastrointestinal epithelium further complicates the issue. Gastrointestinal epithelium occurs in large, broad, flat sheets that may be folded over. The sheets are composed of mucin-producing cells that have uniform nuclear sizes and shapes and well-defined cytoplasmic borders. A luminal border is seen along one or more edges. If smeared with force, the gastrointestinal epithelium may also appear quite dyshesive. Goblet cells and rosettes corresponding to the openings of the crypts of Lieberkühn are two features of intestinal epithelium that will help in this differential diagnosis. Neoplastic epithelium from MCNs usually demonstrates some architectural atypia, such as pseudoacinar formation or papillarity, but minimal nuclear atypia. However, not all sheets from MCNs show atypia, and caution should be exercised when interpreting mucinous epithelium in an aspirate obtained by EUS.

Finally, peripancreatic or retroperitoneal cysts thought to be pancreatic on the basis of imaging studies may present a diagnostic challenge if this possibility is not considered, as occurred with the case of GIST described in the section on peripancreatic cysts. Reported cases are listed in Table 6-3 [14, 95, 102]. In some cases, the cytology has been diagnostic, but others have produced nondiagnostic smears. The cytopathologist may not recognize a diagnostic sample if limited to classifying the neoplasm as a pancreatic cyst.

Caveats in cytologic analysis that will prevent some of these pitfalls include the following:

1. Pseudocyst is a diagnosis of exclusion.
2. Any epithelium present in a cyst fluid aspirate needs explanation.
3. Use special stains that react to mucin to search for background mucin, mucin-containing histiocytes, and mucinous epithelium.
4. Be wary of normal gastrointestinal epithelium.
5. Recommend aspiration of solid areas.
6. Beware of pancreatic cysts that are not really pancreatic in origin.

Although a large number of entities are included in the differential diagnosis of pancreatic cysts, the real crux of the problem in pancreatic cyst fluid analysis is distinguishing pseudocysts from cystic neoplasms, particularly from MCNs. The information presented thus far may be used to formulate an approach to the cytologic evaluation of pancreatic cyst fluids that addresses this problem. The first questions to ask when evaluating a cytology sample from a pancreatic cyst fluid are "What types of cells are present, if any? Are they normal pancreatic elements, contaminants, inflammatory, mucinous or nonmucinous cyst-lining epithelium, or malignant?" A specific diagnosis may be rendered when diagnostic cyst lining or neoplastic cells are present. Care must be taken to avoid interpreting gastrointestinal epithelium as indicative of an MCN. Inflammatory cells alone are a nonspecific finding; however, an infiltrate composed almost exclusively of numerous neutrophils is suggestive of a secondary pancreatic infection, although correlation with clinical and microbiologic studies is necessary. Mucin stains are recommended when the specimen is acellular or the specimen is composed of only histiocytes with few other inflammatory cells, normal pancreatic elements, metaplastic cells, or contaminants other than gastrointestinal epithelium. Mucin stains may also be helpful when the presence of mucinous epithelium is questionable. This approach is summarized in Figure 6-82.

CYST FLUID ANALYSIS OF VISCOSITY, ENZYMES, AND TUMOR MARKERS

Analyzing cyst fluid for viscosity, enzyme levels, isoenzymes, and tumor marker levels may in some cases be a useful aid in the preoperative diagnosis of pancreatic cystic lesions. The cyst fluid markers currently used routinely are shown in Table 6-4 [104–106]. The cyst fluid from mucinous neoplasms can often be recognized by its high viscosity [104]. Pancreatic enzymes, such as amylase, lipase, and amylase isoenzymes, are of limited utility in the differential diagnosis of pancreatic cystic fluids. Amylase and lipase levels are typically elevated in pseudocysts and are usually lower in neoplasms, particularly SCA, but may be elevated in cystic neoplasms. Isoenzymes, which include P1 and P2 (pancreatic) and S1 (salivary) types, may distinguish between pseudocysts and cystic neoplasms because pseudocysts contain a prominent P1 and P2 peak but cystic neoplasms exhibit a combination of P1 and S1 isoenzymes. Isoenzymes are measured by electrophoresis, a technique that is not widely available and is difficult to interpret, presenting a drawback in the use of these measurements. Leukocyte esterase is the final enzyme marker that has been studied, most useful for the distinction of pseudocyst from SCA.

Tumor markers measured include CEA, CA 72-4, CA 15-3, CA 19-9, CA 125 and tissue polypeptide antigen (TPA). CEA effectively identifies mucinous neoplasms because its level is elevated in mucinous neoplasms and low in other neoplasms and pseudocysts, but measuring CEA is not specific enough to distinguish low-grade MCN from malignant neoplasms. CEA levels need to be interpreted with caution because they have been elevated in mesenteric inclusion cysts and in an enteric duplication cyst [44, 104], leading to a spurious suspicion for MCN. CA 72-4, CA 15-3, and TPA are reportedly specific for malignant pancreatic cysts [104, 105]. Some authors [106] have reported CA 19-9 to aid in the distinction of mucinous tumors from pseudocysts and SCAs, but CA 19-9 has not proven effective in our hands [104]. CA 125, although not specific may be helpful in the distinction of pseudocysts from SCA because its level is not elevated in pseudocysts but is variably elevated in SCA [104].

None of these markers have been approved for this use by the Food and Drug Administration [104]. Furthermore, measurements of tumor marker and enzyme levels need to be standardized within each institution because numeric values obtained with commercial assays vary considerably [104]. Although these markers add significant information to the interpretation of cyst fluids, cytology remains an essential part of the analysis and is the gold standard.

Pitfalls in the chemical analysis of cyst fluids include direct communication with the pancreatic duct [104], cases of nonpancreatic "pancreatic" cysts, and cyst fluid to which normal saline has been added to increase the total volume for processing. Communication of a cystic tumor with a pancreatic duct may lead to washout or contamination of the fluid. Nonpancreatic cysts produce very low enzyme levels. If the cyst fluid is diluted, the volume of the cyst fluid and the volume of normal saline added to it should be recorded and enzyme and tumor marker level measurements adjusted accordingly, if necessary. Cyst fluid analysis is most reliable when a panel of tests is used and the results are internally consistent.

A final caution is that cyst fluid analyses may be diagnostic of that particular fluid but may not represent the complete picture. This occurs when a pseudocyst or retention cyst develops secondary to duct obstruction from either a solid or cystic neoplasm or when cystic neoplasms occur synchronously with other neoplasms. Aspiration of solid areas adjacent to the cyst or aspiration of multiple loculi with separate analysis of the cyst fluid from each loculus circumvents these problems. The appearance of a pseudocyst may antedate the appearance of an obstructing lesion. Therefore, in a patient without any clinical explanation for the development of a pseudocyst, an obstructing pancreatic mass should be excluded. Cooperation among the radiologist, clinician, and pathologist ensures aspiration of all significant areas, helps to exclude the possibility of radiologically inapparent entities, and leads to a better understanding and interpretation of all the findings.

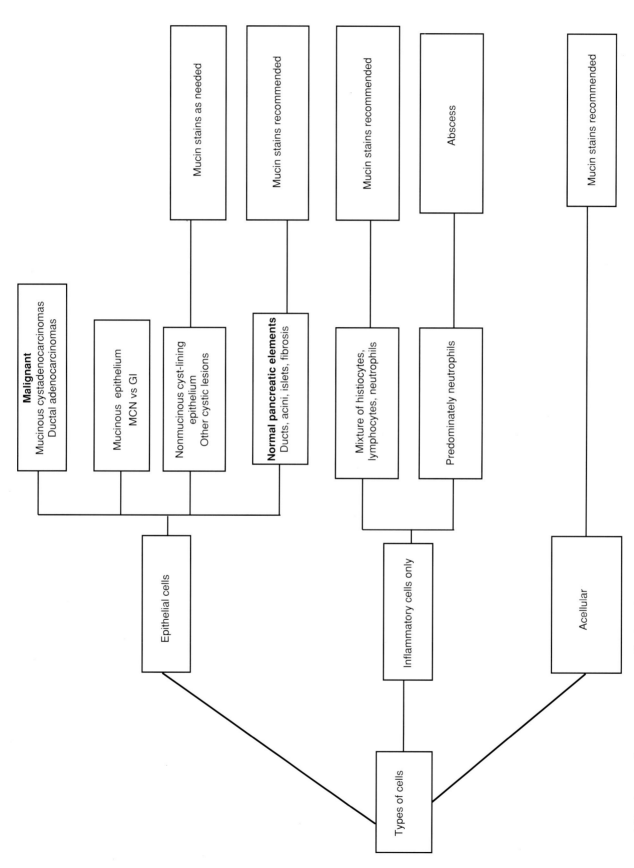

Figure 6-82. Approach to pancreatic cyst fluid cytology. (MCN = mucinous cystic neoplasm; GI = gastrointestinal.)

TABLE 6-4. Cyst Fluid Markers

Parameter	Pseudocyst	Serous Cystadenoma	Mucinous Cystic Neoplasm	Mucinous Cystadenocarcinoma
Cytology	Inflammatory	Glycogenated epithelium	Mucinous epithelium	Malignant cells
Tumor markers				
CEA	Low	Low	High	High
CA 15-3	Low	Low	Low	High
CA 72-4	Low	Low	Low	High
CA 125	Low	Variable	Variable	High
CA 19-9	Low	Low	High	High
TPA	Low	Intermediate	Intermediate	High
Enzymes: amylase or lipase	High	Low	Variable	Variable
Viscosity	Low	Low	High	High

CEA = carcinoembryonic antigen; TPA = tissue polypeptide antigen.

Sources: Data from K Lewandrowski, J Lee, J Southern, et al. Cyst fluid analysis in the differential diagnosis of pancreatic cysts: a new approach to the preoperative assessment of pancreatic cyst lesions. AJR Am J Roentgenol 1995;164:815; and JM Yang, JF Southern, AL Warshaw, et al. Proliferation tissue polypeptide antigen distinguishes malignant mucinous cyst adenocarcinomas from benign cystic tumors and pseudocysts. Am J Surg 1996;171:126.

Some final caveats to observe when analyzing pancreatic cyst fluids include the following:

1. Use a panel of tests.
2. Consider the possibility of another process, such as an obstructing mass, if the cytologic findings are not consistent with the clinical presentation.
3. Cooperation among the cytologists, radiologists, clinicians, and endoscopists is advocated for best interpretation of the results.

The techniques used to prepare pancreatic cyst fluids for cytology and analysis of enzymes and tumor markers are described in Chapter 9.

REFERENCES

1. Cubilla AL, Fitzgerald PJ (eds). Cysts. In Tumors of the Exocrine Pancreas (2nd ed). Washington, DC: Armed Forces Institute of Pathology, 1984;60.

2. Warshaw AL, Rutledge PL. Cystic tumors mistaken for pancreatic pseudocysts. Ann Surg 1987;205:393.

3. Warshaw AL, Compton CC, Lewandrowski K, et al. Cystic tumors of the pancreas. New clinical radiological and pathologic observations in 67 patients. Ann Surg 1990;212:432.

4. Morohoshi T, Held G, Klöppel G. Exocrine pancreatic tumours and their histological classification. A study based on 167 autopsy and 97 surgical cases. Histopathology 1983;7:645.

5. Lumsden A, Bradley EL III. Pseudocyst or cystic neoplasm? Differential diagnosis and initial management of cystic pancreatic lesions. Hepatogastroenterol 1989;36:462.

6. Sachs JR, Deren JJ, Sohn M, et al. Mucinous cystadenoma: pitfalls of differential diagnosis. Am J Gastroenterol 1989;84:811.

7. Isaacs P, Pinder C, Jourdan M, et al. Therapeutic aspiration of pseudocysts: a cautionary tale of the pancreas. Am J Gastroenterol 1986;81:1087.

8. Lewandrowski KB, Southern JF, Pins MR, et al. Cyst fluid analysis in the differential diagnosis of pancreatic cysts: a comparison of pseudocysts, serous cystadenomas, mucinous cystic neoplasms, and mucinous cystadenocarcinoma. Ann Surg 1993;217:41.

9. Cruikshank AH, Benbow EW. Pathology of the Pancreas (2nd ed). London: Springer-Verlag, 1995.

10. Crowley JJ, McAlister WH. Congenital pancreatic pseudocyst: a rare cause of abdominal mass in a neonate. Pediatr Radiol 1996;26:210.

11. Goulet RJ, Goodman J, Schaffer R, et al. Multiple pancreatic pseudocyst disease. Ann Surg 1984;199:6.

12. D'Egidio A, Schein M. Pancreatic pseudocysts: a proposed classification and its management implications. Br J Surg 1991;78:981.

13. Centeno BA, Lewandrowski KB, Warshaw AL, et al. Cyst fluid cytologic analysis in the differential diagnosis of pancreatic cystic lesions. Am J Clin Pathol 1994;101:483.

14. Centeno BA, Warshaw AL, Mayo-Smith W, et al. Cytological diagnosis of pancreatic cystic lesions: a

prospective study of 28 percutaneous aspirates. Acta Cytol 1997;41:972.

15. Cubilla AL, Fitzgerald PF (eds). Inflammatory Lesions and the Diagnosis of Cancer. In Tumors of the Exocrine Pancreas (Vol 2). Washington, DC: Armed Forces Institute of Pathology, 1984;65.

16. Olurin EO. Pancreatic cysts: a report of 10 cases. Br J Surg 1971;58:502.

17. Frias-Hidvegi D. Cysts of the Pancreas. In Guides to Clinical Aspiration Biopsy: Liver and Pancreas. Tokyo: Igaku-Shoin, 1988;227.

18. Fedorak IJ, Ko TC, Djuricin G, et al. Secondary pancreatic infections: are they distinct clinical entities? Surgery 1992;112:824.

19. Warshaw AL. Pancreatic abscesses. N Engl J Med 1972;287:1234.

20. Richter JM, Jacoby GA, Shapiro RH, et al. Pancreatic abscess due to Candida albicans. Ann Intern Med 1982;97:221.

21. Jorda M, Essenfeld H, Garcia E, et al. The value of fine-needle aspiration cytology in the diagnosis of inflammatory pancreatic masses. Diagn Cytopathol 1992;8:65.

22. Lemmer ER, Krige JE, Price SK, et al. Hydatid cyst in the head of the pancreas with obstructive jaundice [see comments]. J Clin Gastroenterol 1995;20:136.

23. Kattan YB. Hydatid cysts in pancreas. BMJ 1975;27:729.

24. Morton PCG, Terblanche JT, Bornman PC, et al. Obstructive jaundice caused by an intrapancreatic hydatid cyst. Br J Surg 1981;68:474.

25. Arnaud A, Sarles JC, Sahel J, et al. Distal pancreatic atrophy and diabetes associated with an intrapancreatic hydatid cyst. Pancreas 1992;7:394.

26. Hira PR, Shweiki H, Lindberg LG, et al. Diagnosis of cystic hydatid disease: role of aspiration cytology. Lancet 1988;2:655.

27. Filice C, Pirola F, Brunetti E, et al. A new therapeutic approach for hydatid liver cysts. Aspiration and alcohol injection under sonographic guidance. Gastroenterology 1990;98:1366.

28. Nakano I, Miyahara T, Ito T, et al. Giardiasis in pancreas. Lancet 1995;345:524.

29. Auringer ST, Ulmer JL, Sumner TE, et al. Congenital cyst of the pancreas. J Pediatr Surg 1993;28:1570.

30. Howard JM. Cystic neoplasms and true cysts of the pancreas. Surg Clin North Am 1989;69:651.

31. Sperti C, Pasquali C, Costantino V, et al. Solitary true cyst of the pancreas in adults. Report of three cases and review of the literature. Int J Pancreatol 1995;18:161.

32. Mao C, Greenwood S, Wagner S, et al. Case report. Solitary true cyst of the pancreas in an adult. Int J Pancreatol 1992;12:181.

33. Cotran RS, Kumar V, Robbins SL. Robbins Pathologic Basis of Disease (4th ed). Philadelphia: Saunders, 1989;983.

34. Nygaard KK, Stacy LJ. Solitary congenital (dysontogenetic) cyst of the pancreas, report of a case. Arch Surg 1942;45:206.

35. Louredo Méndez AM, Trinchet Hernández M, Munoz-Calero Peregrín A, et al. Quistes verdaderos del páncreas en el adulto. Rev Esp Enferm Dig 1995;87:544.

36. Mares AJ, Hirsch M. Congenital cysts of the head of the pancreas. J Pediatr Surg 1997;12:547.

37. Neumann HPH, Dinkel E, Brambs H, et al. Pancreatic lesions in the von Hippel–Lindau syndrome. Gastroenterology 1991;101:465.

38. Hough DM, Stephens DH, Johnson CD, et al. Pancreatic lesions in von Hippel–Lindau disease: prevalence, clinical significance, and CT findings. AJR Am J Roentgenol 1994;162:1091.

39. Torra R, Alos L, Ramos J, et al. Renal-hepatic-pancreatic dysplasia: an autosomal recessive malformation. J Med Genet 1996;33:409.

40. Kennedy SM, Hashida Y, Malatack JJ. Polycystic kidneys, pancreatic cysts, and cystadenomatous bile ducts in the oral-facial-digital syndrome type I. Arch Pathol Lab Med 1991;115:519.

41. Rizzo RJ, Szucs RA, Turner MA. Congenital abnormalities of the pancreas and biliary tree in adults. Radiographics 1995;15:49.

42. Flaherty MJ, Benjamin DR. Multicystic pancreatic hamartoma: a distinctive lesion with immunohistochemical and ultrastructural study. Hum Pathol 1992;23:1309.

43. Kohzaki S, Fukuda T, Fujimotu T, et al. Case report: ciliated foregut cyst of the pancreas mimicking teratomous tumor. Br J Radiol 1994;67:601.

44. Pins MR, Compton CC, Southern JF, et al. Ciliated enteric duplication cyst presenting as a pancreatic cystic neoplasm: report of a case with cyst fluid analysis. Clin Chem 1992;38:1501.

45. Truong LD, Stewart MG, Hao H, et al. A comprehensive characterization of lymphoepithelial cyst associated with the pancreas. Am J Surg 1995;170:27.

46. Goodman P, Kumar D, Balachandran S. Lymphoepithelial cyst of the pancreas. Abdom Imaging 1994;19:157.

47. Ueno S, Muranaka T, Maekawa S, et al. Radiographic features in lymphoepithelial cyst of the pancreas. Abdom Imaging 1994;19:232.

48. Iacono C, Cracco N, Zamboni G, et al. Lymphoepithelial cyst of the pancreas. Int J Pancreatol 1996;19:71.

49. Rino Y, Morohoshi T, Funo K, et al. Lymphoepithelial cyst of the pancreas: a preoperatively diagnosed case based on an aspiration biopsy. Jpn J Surg 1995;25:1043.

50. Cappellari JO. Fine-needle aspiration cytology of a pancreatic lymphoepithelial cyst. Diagn Cytopathol 1993;9:77.

51. Mitchell ML. Fine needle aspiration biopsy of peripancreatic lymphoepithelial cysts. Acta Cytol 1990;34:462.

52. Markovsky V, Russin VL. Fine-needle aspiration of dermoid cyst of the pancreas: a case report. Diagn Cytopathol 1993;9:66.

53. Assawamatiyanont S, King AD. Dermoid cysts of the pancreas. Am Surg 1977;43:503.

54. Mester M, Trajber HJ, Compton CC, et al. Cystic teratomas of the pancreas. Arch Surg 1990;125:1215.

55. Morohoshi T, Hamamoto T, Kunimura T, et al. Epidermoid cyst derived from an accessory spleen in the pancreas. Acta Pathologica Jpn 1991;41:916.

56. Compagno J, Oertel JE. Microcystic adenomas of the pancreas (glycogen-rich cystadenomas). A clinicopathologic study of 34 cases. Am J Clin Pathol 1978;69:289.

57. Huh JR, Chi JG, Jung KC, et al. Macrocystic serous cystadenoma of pancreas—a case report. J Korean Med Sci 1994;9:78.

58. Lewandrowski K, Warshaw A, Compton C. Macrocystic serous cystadenoma of the pancreas. Hum Pathol 1992;23:871.

59. Yoshimi N, Sugie S, Tanaka T, et al. A rare case of serous cystadenocarcinoma of the pancreas. Cancer 1992;69:2449.

60. George DH, Murphy F, Michalski R, et al. Serous cystadenocarcinoma of the pancreas: a new entity? Am J Surg Pathol 1989;13:61.

61. Ohta T, Nagakawa T, Itoh H, et al. A case of serous cystadenoma of the pancreas with focal malignant changes. Int J Pancreatol 1993;14:283.

62. Kamei K, Funabiki T, Ochiai M, et al. Multifocal pancreatic serous cystadenoma with atypical cells and focal perineural invasion. Int J Pancreatol 1991;10:161.

63. Alpert LC, Truong LD, Bosart MI, et al. Microcystic adenoma (serous cystadenoma) of the pancreas. A study of 14 cases with immunohistochemical and electron-microscopic correlation. Am J Surg Pathol 1988;12:251.

64. Jones EC, Suen KC, Grant DR, et al. Fine-needle aspiration cytology of neoplastic cysts of the pancreas. Diagn Cytopathol 1987;3:238.

65. Young NA, Villani MA, Khoury P, et al. Differential diagnosis of cystic neoplasms of the pancreas by fine-needle aspiration. Arch Pathol Lab Med 1991;115:571.

66. Hittmair A, Pernthaler H, Totsch M, et al. Preoperative fine needle aspiration cytology of a microcystic adenoma of the pancreas. Acta Cytol 1991;35:546.

67. Nguyen GK, Vogelsang PJ. Microcystic adenoma of the pancreas. A report of two cases with fine needle aspiration cytology and differential diagnosis. Acta Cytol 1993;37:908.

68. Compagno J, Oertel JE. Mucinous cystic neoplasms of the pancreas with overt and latent malignancy (cystadenocarcinoma and cystadenoma). Am J Clin Pathol 1978;69:573.

69. Albores-Saavedra J, Gould EW, Angeles-Angeles A, et al. Cystic tumors of the pancreas. Pathol Annu 1990;25(pt. 2):19.

70. Yamaguchi K, Enjoji M. Cystic neoplasms of the pancreas. Gastroenterology 1987;92:1934.

71. Klöppel G, Solcia E, Longnecker DS, et al. Histological Typing of Tumours of the Exocrine Pancreas (2nd ed). Berlin: Springer-Verlag, 1996.

72. Lichtenstein DR, Carr-Locke DL. Mucin-secreting tumors of the pancreas. Gastrointest Endosc Clin N Am 1995;5:237.

73. Santini D, Campione O, Salerno A, et al. Intraductal papillary-mucinous neoplasm of the pancreas. Arch Pathol Lab Med 1995;119:209.

74. Yanagisawa A, Ohashi K, Hori M, et al. Ductectatic-type mucinous cystadenoma and cystadenocarcinoma of the human pancreas: a novel clinicopathological entity. Jpn J Cancer Res 1993;84:474.

75. Kawarada Y, Yano T, Yamamoto T, et al. Intraductal mucin-producing tumors of the pancreas. Am J Gastroenterol 1992;87:634.

76. Uehara H, Nakaizumi A, Iishi H, et al. Cytologic examination of pancreatic juice for differential diagnosis of benign and malignant mucin-producing tumors of the pancreas. Cancer 1994;74:826.

77. Cappellari JO, Geisinger KR. Fine-Needle Aspiration Cytology of Malignant Papillary-Cystic Tumor of the Pancreas. ASCP Cytopathology Check Sample (Vol C91-5). American Society of Clinical Pathologists, 1991.

78. Zinner MJ, Shurbaji MS, Cameron JL. Solid and papillary epithelial neoplasms of the pancreas. Surgery 1990;108:475.

79. Friedman AC, Lichtenstein JE, Fishman EK, et al. Solid and papillary epithelial neoplasm of the pancreas. Radiology 1985;154:333.

80. Bombi JA, Milla A, Badal JM, et al. Papillary-cystic neoplasm of the pancreas. Cancer 1984;54:780.

81. Tait N, Greenberg ML, Richardson AJ, et al. Frantz's tumour: papillary and cystic carcinoma of the pancreas. Aust N Z J Surg 1995;65:237.

82. Ogawa T, Isaji S, Okamura K, et al. A case of radical resection for solid cystic tumor of the pancreas with widespread metastases in the liver and greater omentum. Am J Gastroenterol 1993;88:1436.

83. Miettinen M, Partanen S, Fraki O, et al. Papillary cystic tumor of the pancreas. An analysis of cellular differentiation by electron microscopy and immunohistochemistry. Am J Surg Pathol 1987;11:855.

84. Bondeson L, Bondeson AG, Genell S, et al. Aspiration cytology of a rare solid and papillary epithelial neoplasm of the pancreas. Light and electron microscopic study of a case. Acta Cytol 1984;28:605.

85. Wilson MB, Adams DB, Garen PD, et al. Aspiration cytologic, ultrastructural, and DNA cytometric findings of solid and papillary tumor of the pancreas. Cancer 1992;69:2235.

86. Katz LB, Ehya H. Aspiration cytology of papillary cystic neoplasm of the pancreas [see comments]. Am J Clin Pathol 1990;94:328.

87. Granter SR, DiNisco S, Granados R. Cytologic diagnosis of papillary cystic neoplasm of the pancreas. Diagn Cytopathol 1995;12:313.

88. Buetow PC, Parrino TV, Buck JL, et al. Islet cell tumors of the pancreas: pathologic-imaging correlation among size, necrosis and cysts, calcification, malignant behavior, and functional status. AJR Am J Roentgenol 1995;165:1175.

89. Weissmann D, Lewandrowski K, Godine J, et al. Pancreatic cystic islet-cell tumors. Clinical and pathologic features in two cases with cyst fluid analysis. Int J Pancreatol 1994;15:75.

90. Iacono C, Serio G, Fugazzola C, et al. Cystic islet cell tumors of the pancreas. A clinico-pathological report of two nonfunctioning cases and review of the literature. Int J Pancreatol 1992;11:199.

91. Davtyan H, Nieberg R, Reber HA. Pancreatic cystic endocrine neoplasms. Pancreas 1990;5:230.

92. Thompson NW, Eckhauser FE, Vinik AI, et al. Cystic neuroendocrine neoplasms of the pancreas and liver. Ann Surg 1984;199:158.

93. Cantrell BB, Cubilla AL, Erlandson RA, et al. Acinar cell cystadenocarcinoma of human pancreas. Cancer 1981;47:410.

94. Stamm B, Burger H, Hollinger A. Acinar cell cystadenocarcinoma of the pancreas. Cancer 1987;60:2542.

95. Sperti C, Cappellazzo F, Pasquali C, et al. Cystic neoplasms of the pancreas: problems in differential diagnosis. Am Surg 1993;59:740.

96. Kobayashi H, Tsuyoshi I, Morata R, et al. Pancreatic cavernous hemangioma: CT, MRI, US and angiography characteristics. Gastrointest Radiol 1991,16:307.

97. Hayashi J, Yamashita Y, Kakegawa T, et al. A case of cystic lymphangioma of the pancreas. J Gastroenterol 1994;29:372.

98. Gregory IL. Lymphangioma of pancreas. N Y State J Med 1976;76:289.

99. Fan YC, Shih SL, Yan FS, et al. Cavernous lymphangioma of the pancreas: a case report. Pancreas 1995;11:104.

100. Khandelwal M, Lichtenstein GR, Morris JB, et al. Abdominal lymphangioma masquerading as a pancreatic cystic neoplasm. J Clin Gastroenterol 1995; 20:142.

101. Mangin P, Perret M, Ronjon A. Hémangiome du pancréas. Int J Radiol 1985;66:381.

102. Malhotra R, Evans R, Bhawan J, et al. A malignant gastric leiomyoblastoma presenting as an infected pseudocyst of the pancreas. Am J Gastroenterol 1988; 83:452.

103. Centeno BA, Brugge WR, Warshaw AL, et al. Endoscopic ultrasound guided fine needle aspiration of pancreatic cystic lesions. Mod Pathol 1997;10:32A.

104. Lewandrowski K, Lee J, Southern J, et al. Cyst fluid analysis in the differential diagnosis of pancreatic cysts: a new approach to the preoperative assessment of pancreatic cystic lesions. AJR Am J Roentgenol 1995;164:815.

105. Yang JM, Southern JF, Warshaw AL, et al. Proliferation tissue polypeptide antigen distinguishes malignant mucinous cystadenocarcinomas from benign cystic tumors and pseudocysts. Am J Surg 1996; 171:126.

106. Hammel P, Levy P, Voitot H, et al. Preoperative cyst fluid analysis is useful for the differential diagnosis of cystic lesions of the pancreas. Gastroenterology 1995;108:1230.

Neoplasms of the Exocrine and Endocrine Pancreas

Barbara A. Centeno and
Martha Bishop Pitman

DUCTAL ADENOCARCINOMA

Ductal adenocarcinoma accounts for 80–85% of all pancreatic carcinomas, 90% when the variants are included [1]. The incidence began to rise in the 1930s but has been stable since 1973, remaining at approximately nine cases per 100,000 people since 1988. The male-to-female ratio is 1.3:1.0. It is rare before age 45, but the occurrence rises sharply thereafter [2]. Cigarette smoking is the most prominent and firmly established risk factor [2, 3]. Diet is the next most important risk factor; a high intake of fat, meat, or both has been associated with pancreatic cancer. Lower levels of lycopene and selenium have also been associated with an increased risk [2].

More than 90% of patients present with pain and jaundice [2]. Combined with weight loss, these symptoms are the classic triad for carcinomas of the pancreatic head [2]. Carcinomas of the distal pancreas are typically painless and do not produce jaundice until they metastasize [2]. Pancreatic adenocarcinoma is radiologically difficult to distinguish from chronic pancreatitis (see Chapter 5).

Survival is clearly related to stage of disease and resectability at time of diagnosis. The most current tumor-node-metastasis (TNM) staging system used at the Massachusetts General Hospital (MGH) is outlined in Table 7-1, and the stage groupings are outlined in Table 7-2.

The goals of preoperative staging are to identify tumors that are potentially resectable, tumors that are still localized but not resectable, and tumors that have already metastasized to distant sites [2]. The preoperative staging procedure includes peritoneal laparoscopy with peritoneal washings to evaluate for the presence of distant and peritoneal metastases, angiography to assess vascular invasion, and radiologic studies to assess tumor size and extent and metastatic deposits 2 cm or greater in size. If one or more preoperative tests yield positive results (i.e., vascular invasion, extension beyond the pancreas, or metastases), only 5% of the tumors are resectable. If the results of all three tests are negative, 78% are fully resectable [2]. Another contraindication to surgical resection is gross nodal involvement. This type of staging procedure spares patients unnecessary operations. Patients with unresectable neoplasms usually require some form of palliation, such as biliary bypass.

Five-year survival rates after resection of pancreatic carcinomas range from 17% to 24% [2, 4, 5]. Nodal status is an important predictor of survival after resection: Patients with a pN1a nodal status have a 5-year survival of approximately 30%; those with a pN1b nodal status have a 0% 5-year survival rate [6]. The overall 5-year survival rate for all carcinomas is 3–5% [7].

Most pancreatic cancers occur in the head. They are typically poorly delineated and firm, with a tan-yellow cut surface (Figure 7-1). The histomorphology is characterized by neoplastic cells in tubules or glands or singly infiltrating a hyalinized, fibrous stroma. They are graded as well differentiated, moderately differentiated, and poorly differentiated, according to the World Health Organization classification (Figures 7-2 to 7-4) [1]. Histologic grading correlates with stage at presentation and prognosis [1]. Variants discussed in individual sections of this chapter include adenosquamous carcinoma, mucinous noncystic carcinoma, and signet-ring cell carcinoma.

TABLE 7-1. Tumor-Node-Metastasis Staging System

Tumor size

T0	No evidence of tumor
Tis	Carcinoma in situ
T1	Tumor ≤2 cm, limited to pancreas
T2	Tumor >2 cm, limited to pancreas
T3	Tumor extends into duodenum, bile duct, and/or peripancreatic tissues
T4	Tumor extends into stomach, spleen, colon, and/or large vessels

Regional lymph nodes

N0	Regional lymph node metastases absent
N1	Regional lymph node metastases present
N1a	Metastasis to a single regional lymph node
N1b	Metastasis in multiple regional lymph nodes

Distant metastasis

M0	No distant metastasis
M1	Distant metastasis

Source: Adapted from ID Fleming, JS Cooper, DE Henson, et al, eds. AJCC Cancer Staging Manual (5th ed). Philadelphia: Lippincott-Raven, 1997.

TABLE 7-2. Staging Systems

Stage	I	N	M
Stage 0	Tis	N0	M0
Stage I	T1,T2	N0	M0
Stage II	T3	N0	M0
Stage III	T1–T3	N1	M0
Stage IVA	T4	Any N	M0
Stage IVB	Any T	Any N	M1

Source: ID Fleming, JS Cooper, DE Henson, et al, eds. AJCC Cancer Staging Manual (5th ed). Philadelphia: Lippincott-Raven, 1997.

The reported sensitivity of pancreatic fine needle aspiration biopsy (FNAB) for the diagnosis of ductal adenocarcinoma varies from 50% to 100% [8–20], but the specificity is usually 100% [8–20]. The reported positive predictive values are 92–100% [12, 14, 15, 18], the negative predictive value is 55.6% [12], and the reported overall accuracy is 80% [18].

Only one study has objectively evaluated cytologic grading of pancreatic adenocarcinomas [21]. Using Black's nuclear grading system developed for breast cancer, this study evaluated nuclear size, membrane shape, chromatin content, and presence or absence of nucleoli to grade the pancreatic adenocarcinomas as well, moderately, or poorly differentiated. Cytologic nuclear grading was shown to have significant impact on prediction of patient survival.

At MGH, percutaneous FNAB of potentially resectable pancreatic neoplasms is performed only when necessary after low-dose radiation [2] to avoid peritoneal dissemination of tumor cells. However, potentially resectable pancreatic neoplasms are now being aspirated at the MGH under endoscopic ultrasound guidance because this eliminates the potential of peritoneal dissemination (see Chapter 3).

Well-Differentiated Adenocarcinoma

The cellularity of FNAB smears varies, with six neoplastic groups being the minimum number recommended for the diagnosis (Figure 7-5) [20].

Well-differentiated adenocarcinomas tend to be more cohesive than higher-grade ductal carcinomas, with minimal nuclear alterations [20]. The sheets and groups of malignant cells are typically thick because of nuclear crowding and overlapping, and they may appear very tightly cohesive around the edges due to a lack of peripheral dyshesion (Figure 7-6) [20]. Some well-differentiated adenocarcinomas have abundant cytoplasmic mucin, which imparts an exaggerated honeycomb appearance to the sheets (Figure 7-7). The degree of nuclear atypia and irregularity is much less than in the higher-grade carcinomas. Instead of coarse nuclear chromatin, patchy chromatin clearing is a more constant finding (Figure 7-8). Extreme convolutional deformities of the nuclei are less frequently found. Instead, more subtle nuclear irregularities (Figure 7-9) and pyramidal or carrot-shaped nuclei are more common (Figure 7-10). Necrosis and mitotic activity may be present, but to a smaller extent (Figure 7-11).

FIGURE 7-1. Ductal adenocarcinoma. Whipple resection specimen showing ill-defined, white, firm mass with stellate borders in the head of the pancreas (*arrows*).

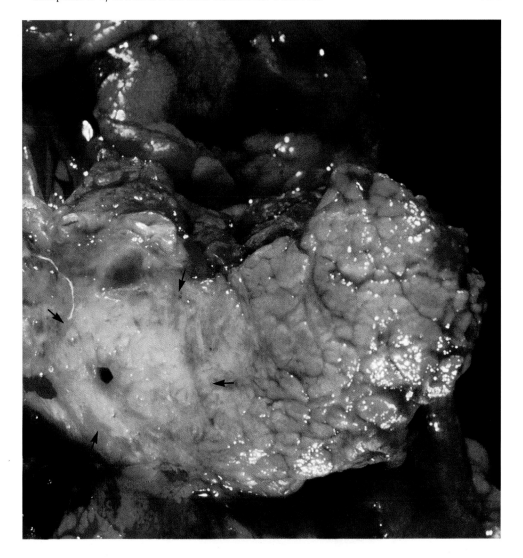

FIGURE 7-2. Ductal adenocarcinoma, well differentiated. Histology slide showing a gland with irregular contours infiltrating a desmoplastic stroma. The nuclei are basally located and show minimal cytologic atypia. The nuclear-to-cytoplasmic ratio is low (Hematoxylin and Eosin, 40×).

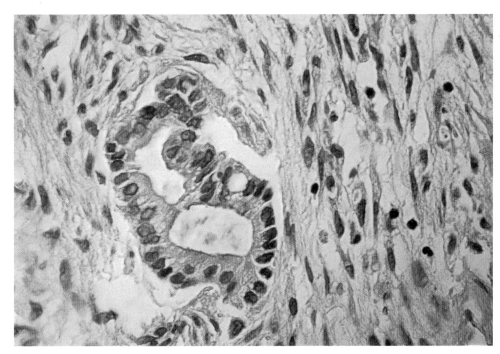

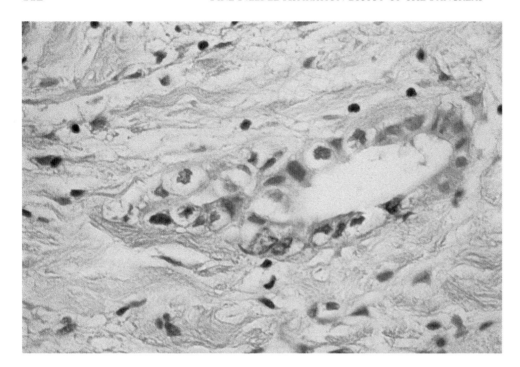

FIGURE 7-3. Ductal adeno-carcinoma, moderately differentiated. An irregularly shaped malignant gland infiltrates a desmoplastic stroma. The cells have abundant clear cytoplasm due to mucin production. The nuclei have lost their polarity and show nuclear membrane irregularities and hyperchromasia. The nuclear-to-cytoplasmic ratio is increased (Hematoxylin and Eosin, 40×).

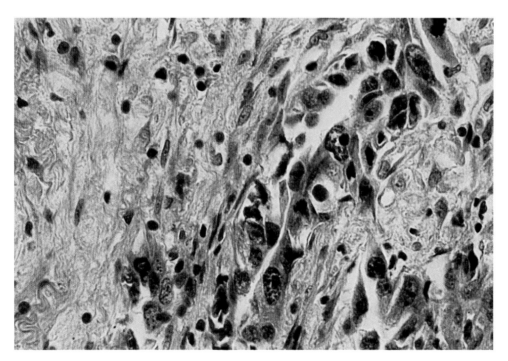

FIGURE 7-4. Ductal adeno-carcinoma, poorly differentiated. The carcinoma is composed of single cells and dyshesive nests. The malignant cells have a very high nuclear-to-cytoplasmic ratio and marked nuclear pleomorphism, nuclear hyperchromasia, nuclear membrane irregularities, and prominent nucleoli. A mitotic figure is evident (Hematoxylin and Eosin, 40×; ×1.6 optivar).

FIGURE 7-5. Ductal adeno-carcinoma, well differenti-ated. Low-power view of a fine needle aspiration biopsy smear showing a very cellular smear with numerous groups of malig-nant cells (Hematoxylin and Eosin, 10×).

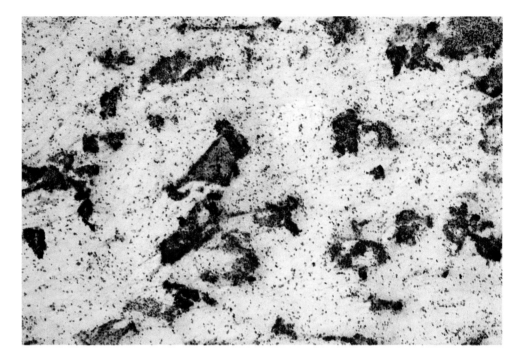

FIGURE 7-6. Ductal adeno-carcinoma, well differenti-ated. Cohesive group of malignant cells with extreme nuclear overlap-ping and crowding and a cribriform space. The periphery of the group is smooth and lacks feather-ing (Papanicolaou, 40×).

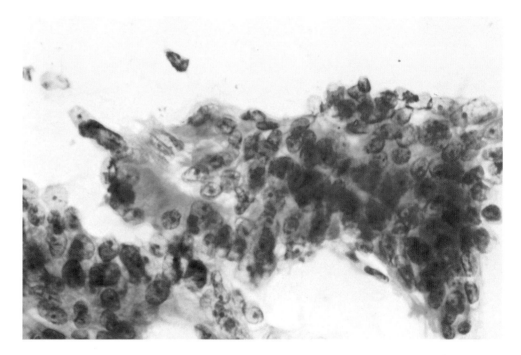

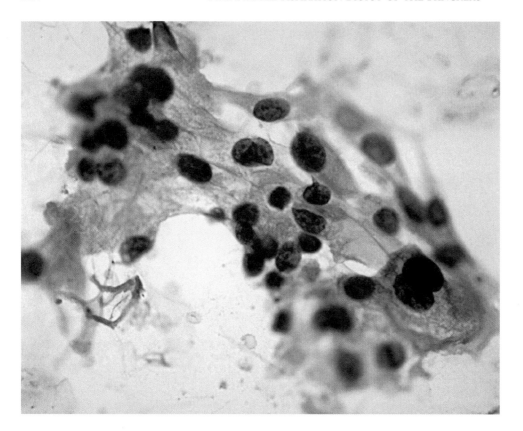

FIGURE 7-7. Ductal adeno-carcinoma, well differenti-ated. Slightly dyshesive sheet of neoplastic epithe-lium with an exaggerated honeycomb appearance due to the presence of abundant cytoplasmic mucin. The cytoplasmic borders are sharply defined. The nuclei are enlarged, hyperchro-matic, and only slightly irregular in shape (Hema-toxylin and Eosin, 40×; ×1.25 optivar).

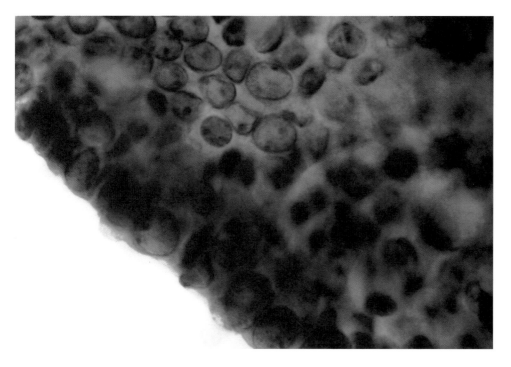

FIGURE 7-8. Ductal adeno-carcinoma, well differenti-ated. The nuclei are pale, with parachromatin clear-ing (Papanicolaou, 100×; ×1.25 optivar).

FIGURE 7-9. Ductal adeno-carcinoma, well differenti-ated. Crowded, overlapping sheet of malignant cells. The nuclei show slight indentations, notches, and grooves but no extreme convolutional deformities. The nucleoli are prominent and the chromatin is pale (Papanicolaou, 63×).

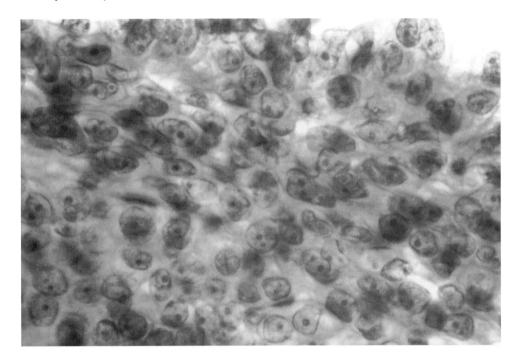

FIGURE 7-10. Ductal ade-nocarcinoma, well differen-tiated. Sheet of neoplastic cells with pyramidal, car-rot-shaped nuclei, some of which have pointed ends. Also seen is a mitotic figure (Hematoxylin and Eosin, 40×).

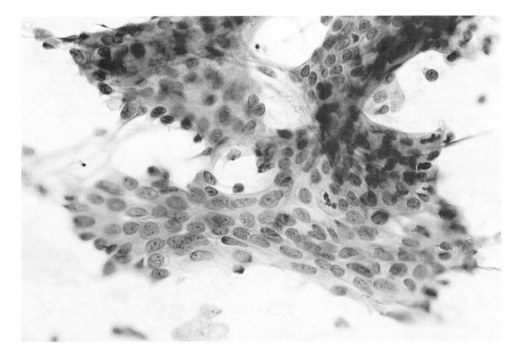

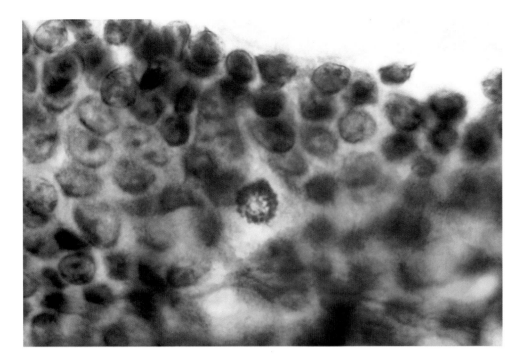

FIGURE 7-11. Ductal adenocarcinoma, well differentiated. Prominent mitotic figure (Papanicolaou, 100×; ×1.6 optivar).

Cytology of Well-Differentiated Adenocarcinoma

- Cohesive clusters or exaggerated honeycombed sheets
- ± Cytoplasmic mucin
- Pyramidal or carrot-shaped nuclei
- Parachromatin clearing
- Scant dyshesion, mitoses, or necrosis

See Chapter 5 for a more detailed discussion of reactive epithelial changes and malignancy.

Moderately Differentiated Adenocarcinoma

Moderately differentiated adenocarcinomas are more easily recognized as malignant. The cellularity of smears is generally high. An exaggerated honeycomb appearance, resulting from abundant cytoplasmic mucin, may also be seen in this grade (Figure 7-12). The sheets also show nuclear crowding but are more dyshesive than well-differentiated adenocarcinomas along the periphery. Single cells are more easily found (Figure 7-13). The nuclear membrane abnormalities are easily found and include nuclear membrane notching and convolution (Figure 7-14), nuclear hyperchromasia, and coarse chromatin (Figure 7-15). Necrosis and mitotic figures are more easily found (Figure 7-16).

Cytology of Moderately Differentiated Adenocarcinoma

- Three-dimensional groups, exaggerated honey-combed sheets, single cells
- ± Cytoplasmic mucin

- Nuclear membrane convolutions and indentations, "popcorn" nuclei
- Hyperchromasia and coarse chromatin
- Prominent macronucleoli
- Mitoses and necrosis

Poorly Differentiated Adenocarcinoma

Poorly differentiated carcinomas show less glandular differentiation and typically show focal to no mucin production. The cells are typically very dyshesive and occur in small loose groups or as single cells. The degree of nuclear convolutions and atypia is extreme, and mitoses and extensive necrosis with tumor ghost cells are common features (Figures 7-17 to 7-19).

Cytology of Poorly Differentiated Adenocarcinoma

- Mostly single cells and small, loose groups
- Scant cytoplasmic mucin
- Marked nuclear membrane irregularities and hyperchromasia
- Abundant necrosis and mitoses

Variants of Ductal Carcinoma

Adenosquamous Carcinoma

Adenosquamous is the most common variant, accounting for 3–4% of all pancreatic carcinomas [1]. It is defined as a carcinoma composed of neoplastic glandular and squamoid elements in which the squamoid component

FIGURE 7-12. Ductal adenocarcinoma, moderately differentiated. Sheet of neoplastic cells with an exaggerated honeycomb appearance. The nuclei in this sheet, in contrast to those in Figure 7-7, have more obvious features of malignancy (Papanicolaou, 100×).

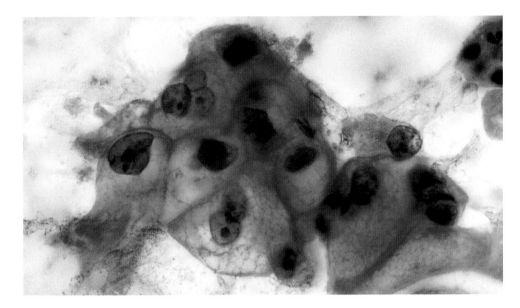

FIGURE 7-13. Ductal adenocarcinoma, moderately differentiated. Cluster of crowded, neoplastic epithelium with peripheral dyshesion and single cells (Papanicolaou, 40×; ×1.6 optivar).

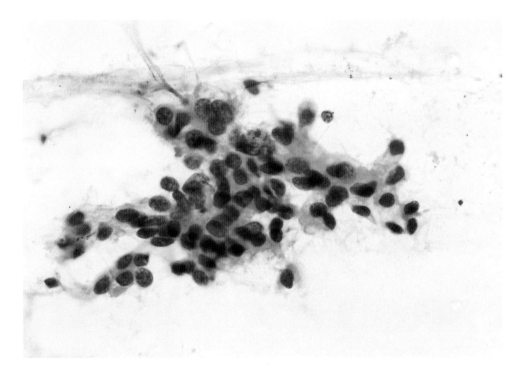

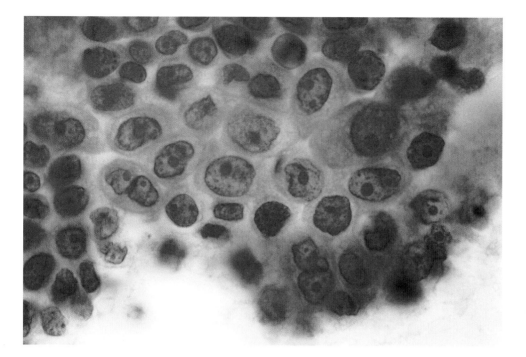

FIGURE 7-14. Ductal adenocarcinoma, moderately differentiated. Significant anisocytosis, nuclear enlargement, and nuclear membrane irregularities are seen, including notches and convolutions. The cells also have prominent nucleoli (Hematoxylin and Eosin, 100×).

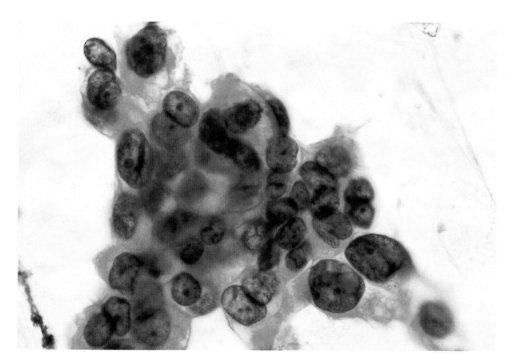

FIGURE 7-15. Ductal adenocarcinoma, moderately differentiated. Coarse chromatin, irregularly distributed in a sheet of neoplastic epithelium from a moderately differentiated adenocarcinoma (Papanicolaou, 100×).

FIGURE 7-16. Ductal ade-
nocarcinoma, moderately
differentiated. Abundant
necrosis in the form of
tumor ghost cells (Papanicolaou, 40×).

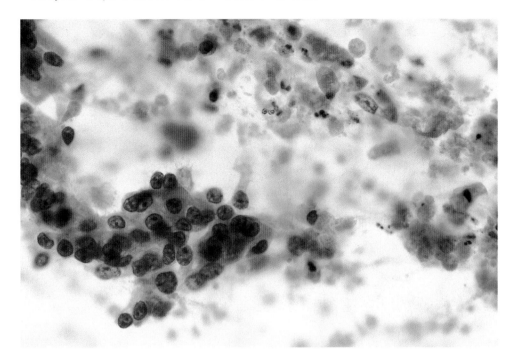

FIGURE 7-17. Ductal ade-
nocarcinoma, poorly differentiated. Low-power
magnification showing a
cellular specimen composed
of a dyshesive population
of neoplastic cells with
background necrosis
(Papanicolaou, 40×; ×1.6
optivar).

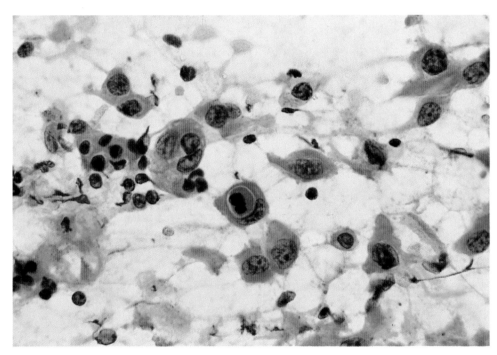

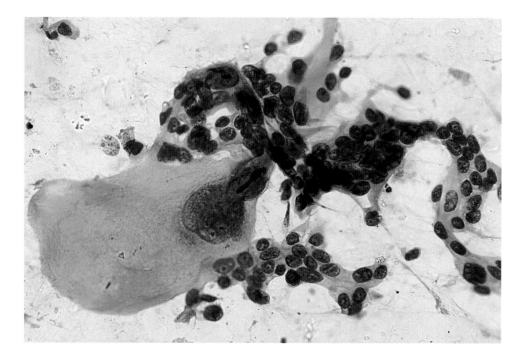

FIGURE 7-18. Ductal adenocarcinoma, poorly differentiated. Single, large cell with a bizarre nucleus and smaller malignant cells in cohesive sheets with scant cytoplasm, and hyperchromatic nuclei with extremely coarse chromatin (Papanicolaou, 40×).

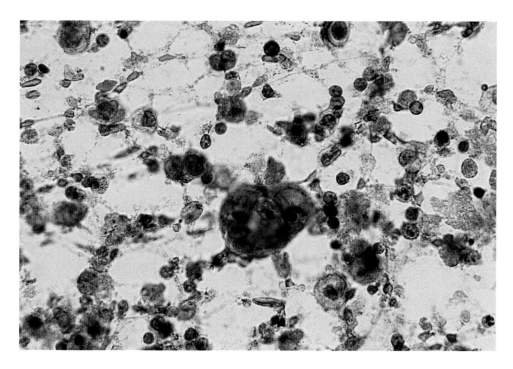

FIGURE 7-19. Ductal adenocarcinoma, poorly differentiated. The malignant cells are arranged in tight groups and have prominent nucleoli. Hemorrhage and necrosis are significant (Papanicolaou, 40×; ×1.6 optivar).

accounts for at least 30% of the tumor [1]. It is thought to develop from metaplasia of a preexisting adenocarcinoma [22]. Pure pancreatic squamous cell carcinoma may occur, but usually, extensive histologic sampling of resected pancreatic carcinomas that initially appear to be pure squamous cell carcinoma reveals a glandular component [1, 23]. Therefore, an extrapancreatic origin should be considered for a pancreatic carcinoma showing only squamous differentiation, keeping in mind that small samples obtained with wedge biopsies, core biopsies, or FNAB may contain only the squamous component in a tumor of otherwise mixed squamous and glandular differentiation. In such cases, although the possibility of a primary pancreatic adenosquamous carcinoma must be considered, metastatic squamous cell carcinoma cannot be excluded [24].

Grossly, these neoplasms resemble the typical ductal adenocarcinoma. Histologically, they have a squa-

FIGURE 7-20. Adenosquamous carcinoma. Cell block showing a single gland of well-differentiated adenocarcinoma surrounded by infiltrating nests of squamous cell carcinoma (Hematoxylin and Eosin, 20×; ×1.6 optivar).

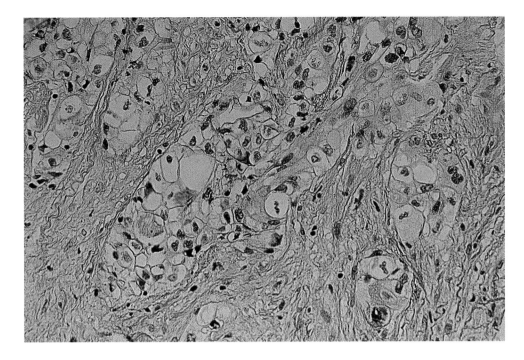

FIGURE 7-21. Adenosquamous carcinoma. Touch preparation of a core showing numerous single cells with dense, eosinophilic cytoplasm and malignant nuclear features (Hematoxylin and Eosin, 63×).

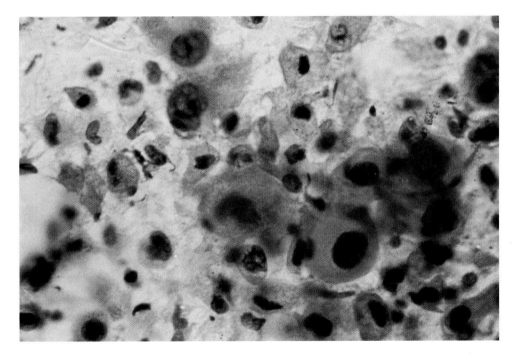

mous component, showing variable differentiation, including keratin production, squamous pearls, and intercellular ridges. The glandular component varies in quantity and differentiation (Figure 7-20).

A few reports have described the FNAB findings [24–26]. The smears are typically very cellular. The proportion of squamous to glandular components varies, as does the degree of differentiation, and in some cases, the squamous component may be the only one identified [24]. The squamous component may occur in sheets or as single cells (Figure 7-21) and may show evidence of cytoplasmic keratinization (Figure 7-22). The glandular component may be readily apparent, but occasionally, single cells with cytoplasmic mucin vacuoles may be the only evidence of glandular differentiation (Figure 7-23).

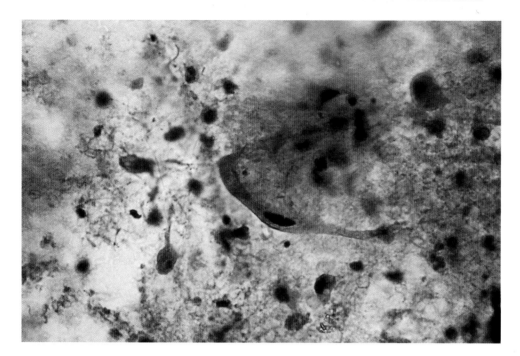

FIGURE 7-22. Adenosquamous carcinoma. Fine needle aspiration biopsy smear showing a single elongated cell with keratinized cytoplasm and abundant background necrosis (Papanicolaou, 63×).

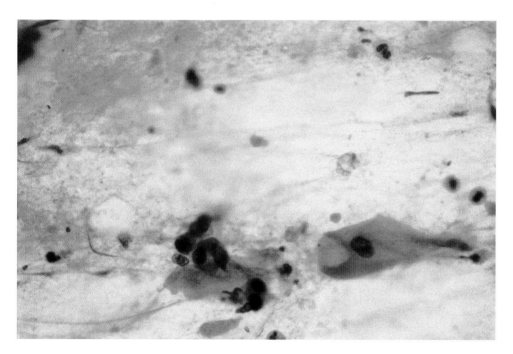

FIGURE 7-23. Adenosquamous carcinoma. Malignant squamous cells and small, single, malignant glandular cells with cytoplasmic vacuoles. These small glandular cells may be the only evidence of glandular differentiation. (Papanicolaou, 100×; ×1.6 optivar).

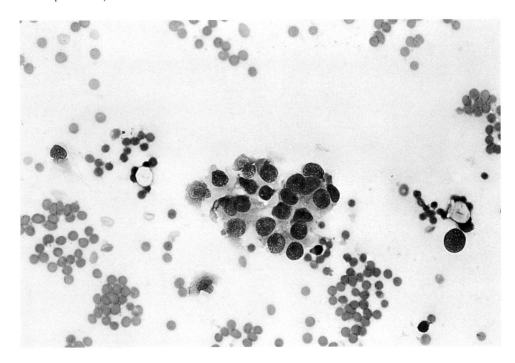

FIGURE 7-24. Mucinous noncystic adenocarcinoma. Sheet of bland cells in a flat, evenly spaced sheet (May-Grünwald–Giemsa, 25×). (Courtesy of Dr. William J. Frable, Virginia Commonwealth University/ Medical College of Virginia School of Medicine, Richmond, VA.)

Cytology of Adenosquamous Carcinoma

- Very cellular
- Squamous component with cytoplasmic keratinization
- Single cells with cytoplasmic mucin vacuoles or sheets showing glandular differentiation

Mucinous Noncystic Carcinoma

The relative frequency of mucinous noncystic carcinoma is 1–2% [1]. The gross cut surface is yellowish white, glistening, and gelatinous, showing many tiny spaces filled with mucoid or creamy material [27]. Histologically, this carcinoma is composed of well-differentiated glands in which more than 50% of the tissue consists of mucin. Microscopically, the neoplasm shows multiloculated pools of mucin with very few cells, either at the rim or floating in the center [27, 28]. This neoplasm may be confused with mucinous cystic neoplasm on cytologic examination. Cytologically, this colloid carcinoma resembles that aspirated from the breast. Sheets of well-differentiated, relatively bland glandular epithelium (Figure 7-24) are admixed with pools of magenta-staining mucin (on Romanowsky stain) (Figure 7-25).

Signet-Ring Cell Carcinoma

The frequency of signet-ring cell carcinoma relative to all pancreatic ductal adenocarcinoma is less than 1% [1]. Signet-ring cells may be found in association with mucinous noncystic adenocarcinoma or mucinous cystadenocarcinomas, and rarely in other types of carcinoma. Histologically, this carcinoma is composed of a dyshesive population of malignant cells diffusely infiltrating the pancreas and containing cytoplasmic mucin vacuoles that compress the nucleus, similar to signet-ring cell carcinomas of the stomach [29].

The smears are very cellular, with numerous single cells showing cytoplasmic mucin vacuoles that distend the cytoplasm and compress and indent the nucleus (Figure 7-26). Background mucin may also be a feature.

Other Variants of Ductal Carcinoma

Other variants include oncocytic carcinoma [29–31], clear cell carcinoma [29, 32], and ciliated cell carcinoma [29, 33]. These are extremely rare and are not included in the World Health Organization classification of pancreatic exocrine neoplasms [1].

OSTEOCLASTIC GIANT CELL TUMOR

Osteoclastic giant cell tumor (OGCT) of the pancreas is a rare primary malignancy of the exocrine pancreas, with only a handful of reports describing its cytologic features on FNAB [34–36].

This tumor was first described by Rosai and found to be morphologically identical to giant cell tumor of bone by light microscopy [37]. Other names given to this tumor include osteoclastoma, giant cell carcinoma, variant of pleomorphic carcinoma, multinuclear giant cell neoplasm, and sarcomatoid carcinoma [38–43]. Mor-

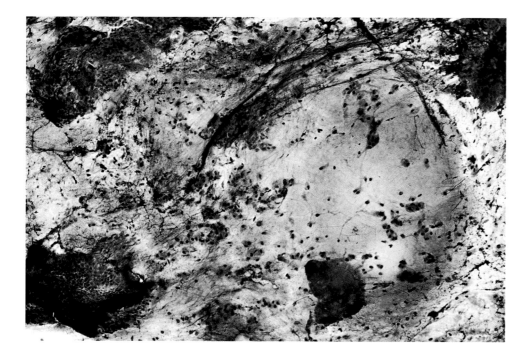

FIGURE 7-25. Mucinous noncystic adenocarcinoma. Sheets of well-differentiated neoplastic glandular epithelium in pools of magenta-colored mucin (May-Grünwald–Giemsa, 10×). (Courtesy of Dr. William J. Frable, Virginia Commonwealth University/Medical College of Virginia School of Medicine, Richmond, VA.)

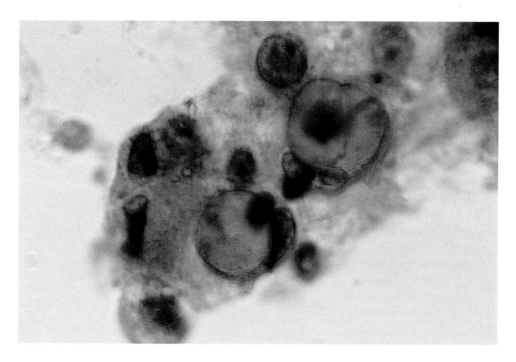

FIGURE 7-26. Signet-ring cell carcinoma. Two signet-ring cells with prominent cytoplasmic mucin vacuoles (Papanicolaou, 100×).

phologically, these tumors closely resemble pleomorphic giant cell carcinoma (PGCC), which is the most important differential diagnosis on cytology and histology [36–39, 43]. OGCT has distinct morphologic features and biological behavior as well as a slightly better prognosis than PGCC. Hybrids of the two tumors have been reported [44].

The histogenesis of the tumor is controversial. Most investigators favor an epithelial origin (as Rosai

originally reported) due to glandular features in some tumors on light microscopy, immunohistochemical studies, and ultrastructural findings [37, 38, 45, 46]. More recent studies, however, support a mesenchymal derivation [36, 38, 44].

OGCTs occur throughout the pancreas in both men and women of various ages, most older than 45 years. The tumors tend to be large (>7 cm), with surgical resection being the treatment of choice [39, 40, 42].

FIGURE 7-27. Osteoclastic giant cell tumor. Osteoclast-type giant cells may dominate the smears (Papanicolaou, 10×).

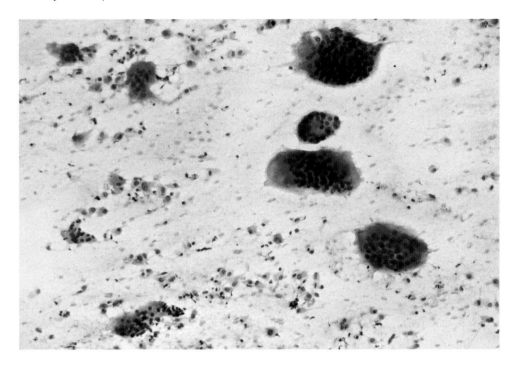

FIGURE 7-28. Osteoclastic giant cell tumor. High-power view of an osteoclast-type giant cell demonstrating centrally clustered, round to oval, overlapping nuclei with bland chromatin and occasional prominent nucleoli, with cyanophilic-staining cytoplasm on Papanicolaou stain (Papanicolaou, 40×).

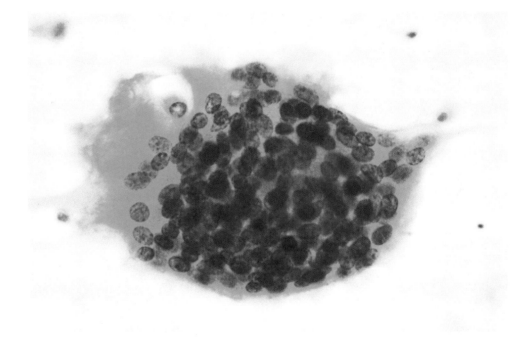

Cytologically, there are three basic cell types: (1) multinucleated osteoclast-type giant cells, (2) epithelioid mononuclear cells, and (3) spindled cells.

Osteoclast-type giant cells frequently dominate the smears (Figure 7-27). These cells are large and contain a variable number of often centrally clustered, round to oval, frequently overlapping nuclei with bland to coarse chromatin and prominent nucleoli. The cytoplasm is abundant, dense, granular and well demarcated, staining cyanophilic with the Papanicolaou stain (Figure 7-28) and deep purple with a Romanowsky stain (Figure 7-29). These cells do not demonstrate mitoses [34, 38].

The mononuclear cells may demonstrate a range of morphologic features, from bland features similar to the giant cells [36] to features that are frankly malignant and consistent with carcinoma (Figures 7-30 to 7-32) [34].

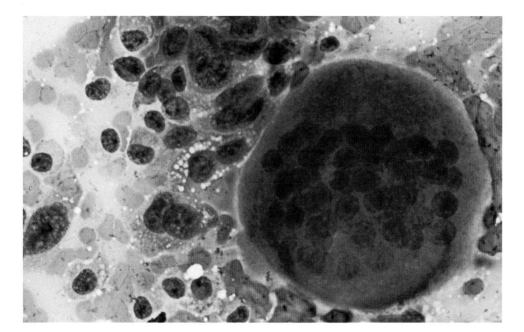

FIGURE 7-29. Osteoclastic giant cell tumor. Large osteoclast-type giant cell associated with mononuclear cells with deep purple–staining cytoplasm on Romanowsky stain (Diff Quik, 40×).

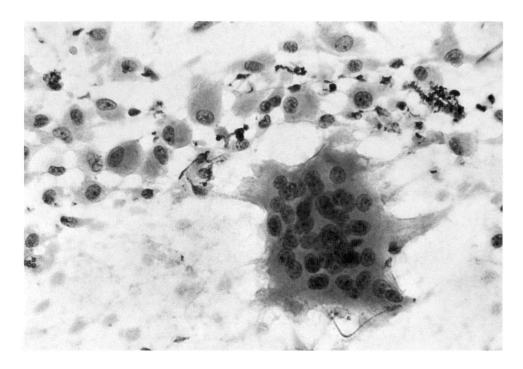

FIGURE 7-30. Osteoclastic giant cell tumor. Bland-appearing mononuclear cells in the company of an osteoclast-type giant cell. The mononuclear cells display eccentric, bland, round nuclei with abundant cytoplasm (Papanicolaou, 25×).

The spindle cells usually demonstrate marked atypicality but may also demonstrate variable degrees of atypia. They may be present singly or in variably cellular, cohesive sheets (Figures 7-33 to 7-35) [35]. Cell blocks can be very helpful in establishing the diagnosis (Figure 7-36).

The primary tumor in the differential diagnosis is PGCC. Although PGCC may contain bland osteoclast-type giant cells, it is distinguished morphologically by the marked pleomorphism and bizarre, anaplastic nature of the vast majority of the mononuclear and multinuclear cells (see below).

Cytology of Osteoclastic Giant Cell Tumor of the Pancreas

- Osteoclast-type giant cells
- Mononuclear cells, with bland or malignant features
- Usually malignant-appearing spindled cells

FIGURE 7-31. Osteoclastic giant cell tumor. Mononuclear cells in an inflammatory background displaying mild to moderate cytologic atypicality (Romanowsky stain, 20×). (Courtesy of Dr. Jan F. Silverman, Allegheny University of the Health Sciences, Medical College of Pennsylvania/Hahnemann School of Medicine, Allegheny General Hospital Campus, Pittsburgh.)

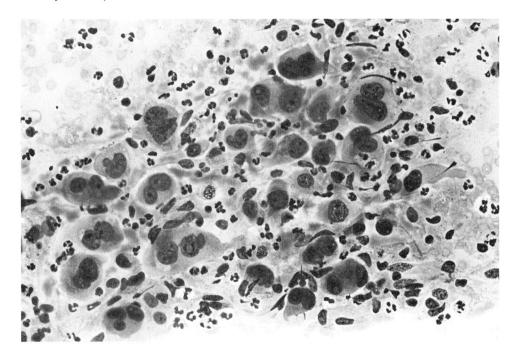

FIGURE 7-32. Osteoclastic giant cell tumor. Malignant-appearing mononuclear cells may be present in some tumors (Romanowsky stain, 40×). (Courtesy of Dr. William J. Frable, Virginia Commonwealth University/Medical College of Virginia School of Medicine, Richmond, VA.)

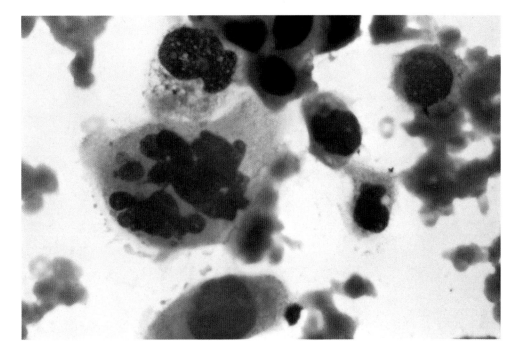

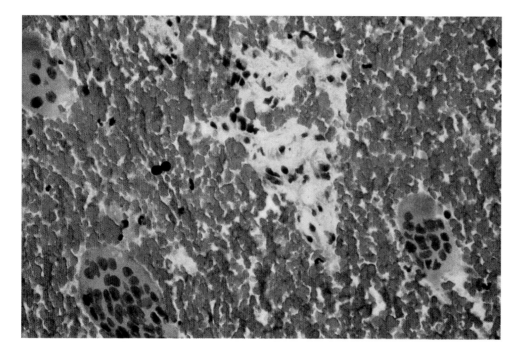

FIGURE 7-33. Osteoclastic giant cell tumor. Osteoclast-type giant cells associated with a fragment of loosely cohesive spindle cells demonstrating moderate atypia (Romanowsky stain, 16×). (Courtesy of Dr. William J. Frable, Virginia Commonwealth University/Medical College of Virginia School of Medicine, Richmond, VA.)

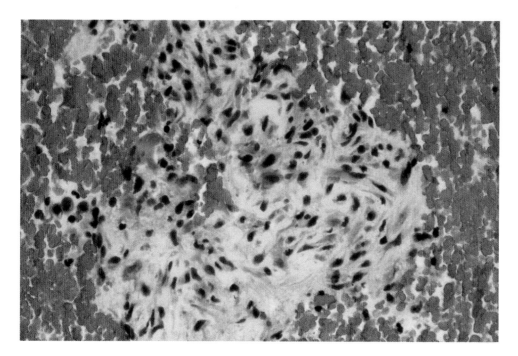

FIGURE 7-34. Osteoclastic giant cell tumor. Cell block preparation demonstrating a fragment of cohesive spindle cells with moderate atypia (Romanowsky stain, 16×). (Courtesy of Dr. William J. Frable, Virginia Commonwealth University/Medical College of Virginia School of Medicine, Richmond, VA.)

FIGURE 7-35. Osteoclastic giant cell tumor. Smears may show highly cellular cohesive fragments of spindle cells admixed with mononuclear cells and osteoclastic giant cells (Papanicolaou, 25×).

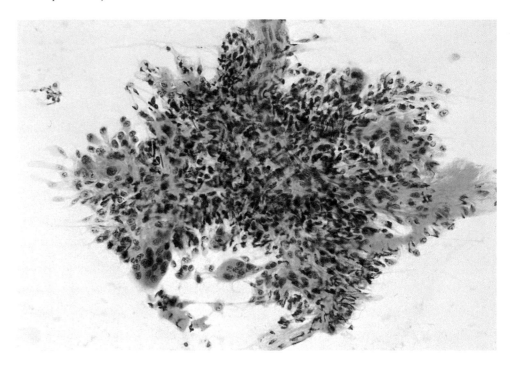

FIGURE 7-36. Osteoclastic giant cell tumor. Cell block preparation demonstrating the association of the bland osteoclast-type giant cells and variably atypical mononuclear cells (Hematoxylin and Eosin, 40×).

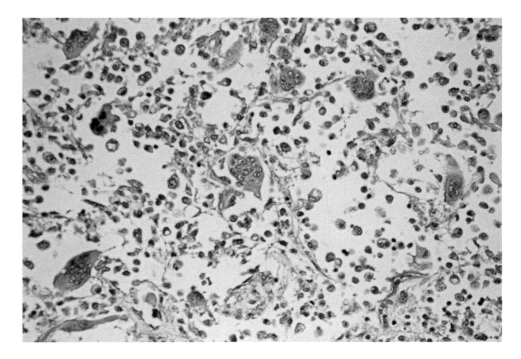

PLEOMORPHIC GIANT CELL CARCINOMA (UNDIFFERENTIATED CARCINOMA)

PGCC of the pancreas, now termed *undifferentiated carcinoma* under the World Health Organization classification [1], is a rare, highly malignant primary tumor of the pancreas first described in 1954 by Sommers and Meissner [47]. Although similar in clinical presentation to the typical pancreatic ductal carcinoma, its biological behavior is more aggressive (survival of 2–3 months vs. survival of 6–8 months), with widespread metastases frequently evident at the time of initial workup [28, 48, 49]. Histologically, the tumor is composed of large, bizarre, anaplastic mononuclear and multinuclear tumor giant cells and malignant spindle cells (Figure 7-37) [28, 40, 48]. Numerous mitotic figures, cytophagocytosis, and vascular invasion are

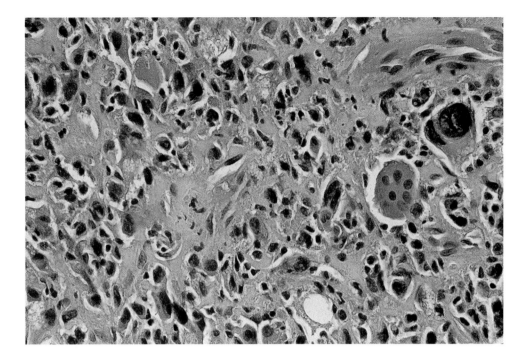

FIGURE 7-37. Pleomorphic giant cell carcinoma. Histologic section showing the marked atypia of the mononuclear cells embedded in a dense sclerotic stroma. Note the lone osteoclast-type giant cell (Hematoxylin and Eosin, 20×).

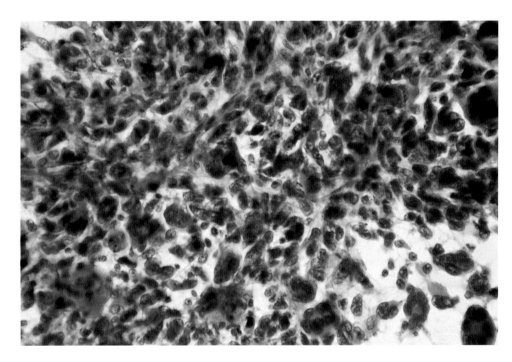

FIGURE 7-38. Pleomorphic giant cell carcinoma. Aspirate smears contain highly cellular but loosely cohesive sheets of large, bizarre, anaplastic malignant cells (Papanicolaou, 40×).

common features [28, 40, 47–49]. These features are uniformly recapitulated on FNAB [39, 50–52], in which a loosely cohesive (Figure 7-38) to noncohesive, dispersed population (Figure 7-39) of large, bizarre, multinucleated (Figure 7-40), mononucleated (Figure 7-41), and spindled cells demonstrate mitotic activity (Figure 7-42) and "cannibalism" (Figure 7-43). Occasionally, a rare osteoclast-type giant cell may also be present (Figure 7-44) [28].

Cytology of Pleomorphic Giant Cell Carcinoma

- Dispersed single-cell population of anaplastic, large, bizarre cells: mononuclear, multinuclear, and spindled
- High mitotic rate
- Cytophagocytosis
- Occasionally rare osteoclast-type giant cells

FIGURE 7-39. Pleomorphic giant cell carcinoma. A highly dispersed, single-cell population may be present (Papanicolaou, 40×).

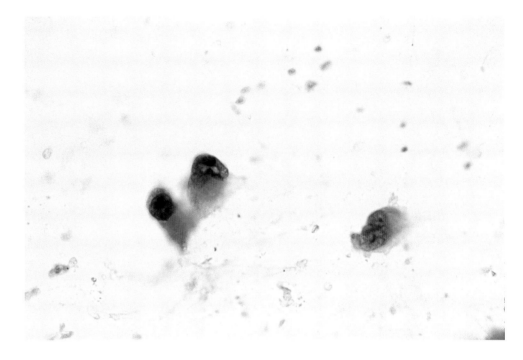

FIGURE 7-40. Pleomorphic giant cell carcinoma. Bizarre multinucleated cells with highly anaplastic, crowded, hyperchromatic, and overlapping nuclei are distinctly different from those seen in the osteoclastic giant cell tumor (Papanicolaou, 40×).

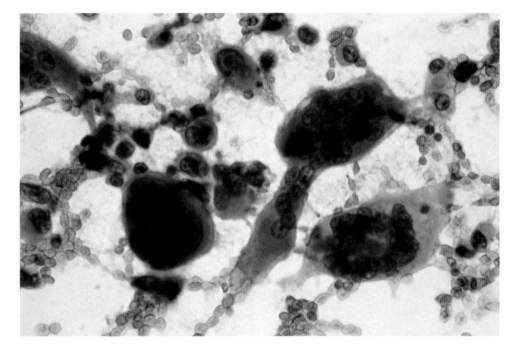

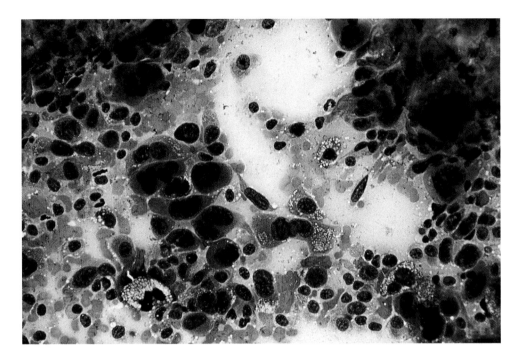

FIGURE 7-41. Pleomorphic giant cell carcinoma. The mononuclear cell population generally appears high grade (Romanowsky stain, 20×).

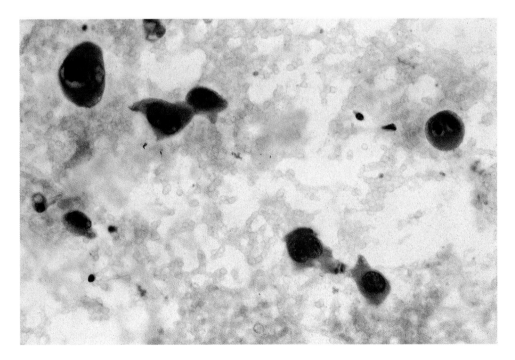

FIGURE 7-42. Pleomorphic giant cell carcinoma. Scattered, bizarre, single mononuclear cells demonstrate a high mitotic rate (Hematoxylin and Eosin, 40×).

FIGURE 7-43. Pleomorphic giant cell carcinoma. "Cannibalism," in which one malignant cell engulfs another, is a feature sometimes encountered in this tumor (Papanicolaou, 40×).

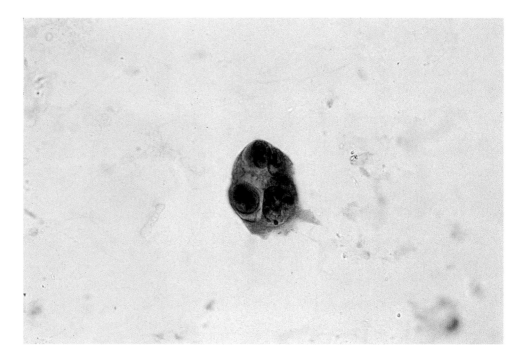

FIGURE 7-44. Pleomorphic giant cell carcinoma. As seen in the histologic section of this tumor (see Figure 7-37), a random osteoclast-type giant cell may be present. This cell type, however, is a minor component of the tumor (Papanicolaou, 40×).

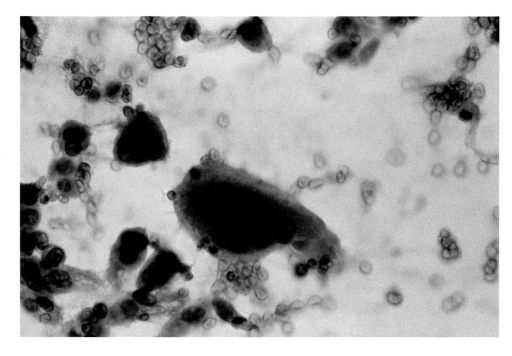

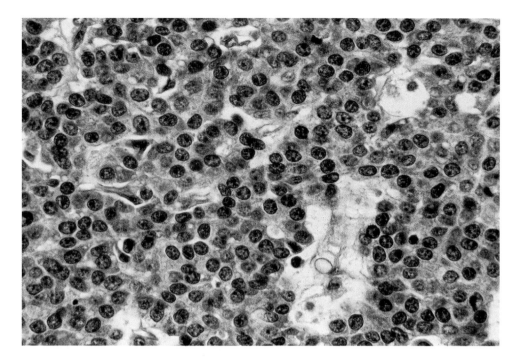

FIGURE 7-45. Acinar cell carcinoma. The histologic hallmark of this tumor at the light microscopic level is the acinar structure, which is generally present in nearly all tumors (Hematoxylin and Eosin, 40×). (Courtesy of Dr. Henry Frierson, University of Virginia School of Medicine, Charlottesville, VA.)

An epithelial origin of this tumor is accepted due to the association of the tumor with foci of obvious adenocarcinoma [28, 40] as well as its epithelial ultrastructural characteristics [45].

Tumors in the differential diagnosis include malignant fibrous histiocytoma, rhabdomyosarcoma, choriocarcinoma, hepatocellular carcinoma, amelanotic melanoma, and metastatic giant cell carcinoma of the lung and thyroid. The diagnosis of OGCT of the pancreas (see previous section) should not be confused with this tumor. Although a rare osteoclastic giant cell may be present in PCA, it is not a dominant feature, as in OGCT.

ACINAR CELL CARCINOMA

Acinar cell carcinoma (ACC) is a rare primary pancreatic neoplasm, with an incidence of 1–2% in most series [53–55] but with an approximately 25% incidence in a recent large study of these tumors [56]. By all accounts, the tumors are highly aggressive, with prognosis and 5-year survival between that of typical ductal carcinoma and islet cell tumor [56]. The overall survival, however, is considerably better than ductal carcinoma, with a 1-year survival rate of more than 50% [56] compared with ductal carcinoma's 1-year survival rate of less than 10% [57].

ACCs are found primarily in white men older than 60 years of age [56] but can be seen in children [56, 58, 59]. Presenting symptoms are nonspecific and, in contrast to ductal carcinoma, generally do not include jaundice. A small percentage of patients with this tumor may present with a syndrome of disseminated fat necrosis and polyarthralgia, a result of serum lipase secretion by the tumor, and a feature associated with a poor prognosis [56, 60–64]. One case report describes the association of ACC and secretion of elastase [65].

Grossly, the tumors are fleshy, circumscribed masses that are occasionally polypoid and cystic [56, 66, 67], with a predilection for the head of the pancreas [68]. Histologically, these tumors are distinctive for their resemblance to normal pancreatic acini. Acinar structures, the light microscopic hallmark of this neoplasm, are generally at least focally present in nearly all tumors (Figure 7-45) [56]. Solid growth may predominate, and trabecular growth patterns often lead to diagnostic difficulty in the distinction from islet cell tumors.

Cytologically, aspirate smears are richly cellular (Figure 7-46), composed of loosely cohesive large and small cell clusters, some in acinar formations (Figure 7-47) and as scattered single cells, many stripped of their cytoplasm (Figure 7-48). The cells resemble normal pancreatic acini, with uniform, minimally pleomorphic cells containing generally euchromatic round to oval, central or eccentric, smooth-contoured nuclei with one or two prominent nucleoli (Figures 7-49 and 7-50). They differ from normal acini, however, in their irregular clustering—acini in smears of normal pancreas have a uniform organoid, grapelike arrangement (Figure 7-51). The cytoplasm is scant to moderate and amphophilic, with

FIGURE 7-46. Acinar cell carcinoma. Aspirate smears are richly cellular and composed of loosely cohesive, large and small cell clusters (Papanicolaou, 25×). (Courtesy of Dr. Henry Frierson, University of Virginia School of Medicine, Charlottesville, VA.)

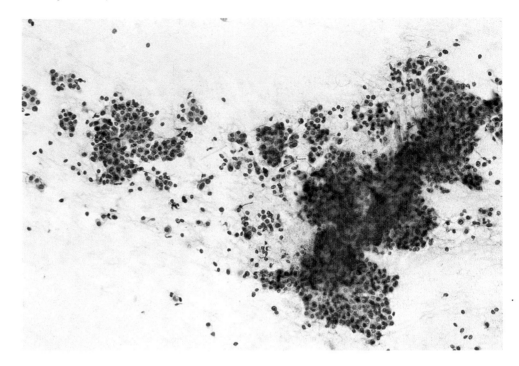

FIGURE 7-47. Acinar cell carcinoma. Acinar formations may be seen focally on aspirate smears (Romanowsky stain, 100×). (Courtesy of Dr. William J. Frable, Virginia Commonwealth University/Medical College of Virginia School of Medicine, Richmond, VA.)

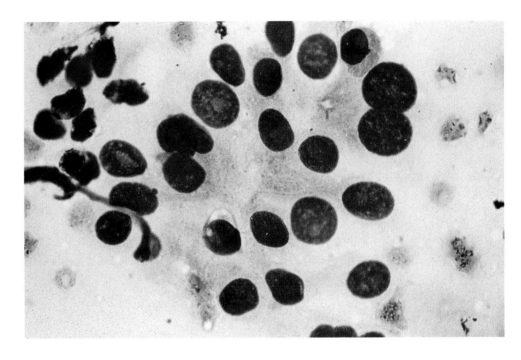

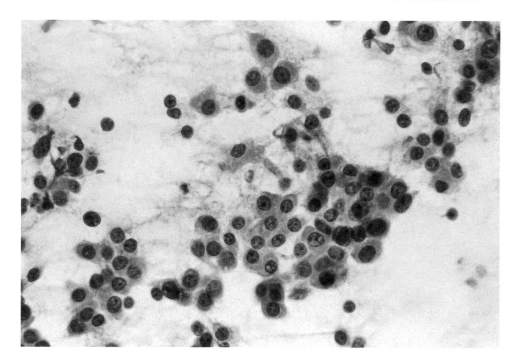

FIGURE 7-48. Acinar cell carcinoma. Single cells may also be present, many of which may be stripped of their cytoplasm, thus yielding a resemblance to lymphocytes (Papanicolaou, 40×). (Courtesy of Dr. Henry Frierson, University of Virginia School of Medicine, Charlottesville, VA.)

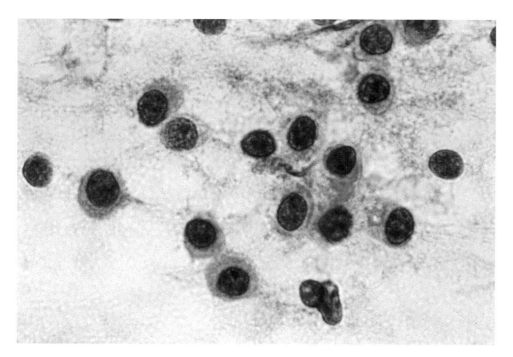

FIGURE 7-49. Acinar cell carcinoma. Individual cells resemble normal acinar epithelial cells with minimally pleomorphic nuclei, a euchromatic chromatin pattern, and one or two small but prominent nucleoli (Papanicolaou, 40×). (Courtesy of Dr. Henry Frierson, University of Virginia School of Medicine, Charlottesville, VA.)

FIGURE 7-50. Acinar cell carcinoma. Romanowsky stain (40×) accentuates cytoplasmic features, showing focal vacuolization of the cells with intact cytoplasm. The nuclear features are less distinct than on Papanicolaou stain. (Courtesy of Dr. Henry Frierson, University of Virginia School of Medicine, Charlottesville, VA.)

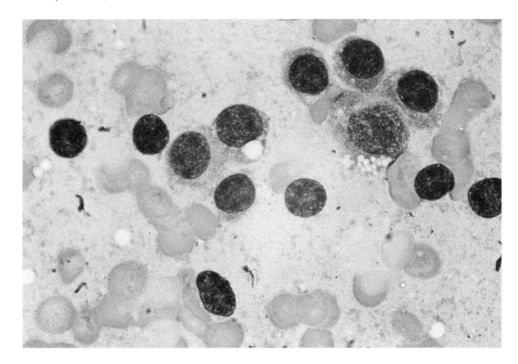

FIGURE 7-51. Normal pancreatic acini. Note the uniform grapelike clusters of the acinar epithelial cells, as opposed to the large and small loosely cohesive sheets and single cells of an acinar cell carcinoma (Papanicolaou, 40×).

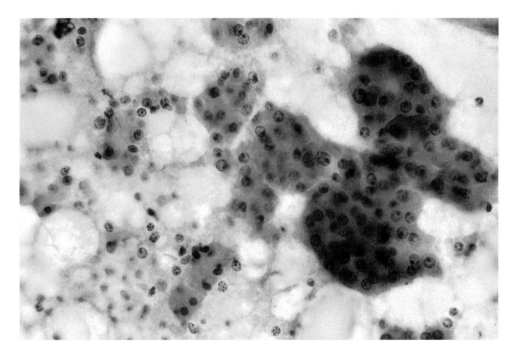

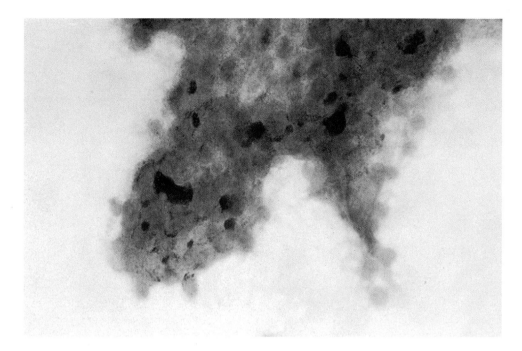

FIGURE 7-52. Acinar cell carcinoma. Periodic acid–Schiff (PAS) stain with diastase digestion accentuates the cytoplasmic granularity (PAS with diastase, 40×). (Courtesy of Dr. Henry Frierson, University of Virginia School of Medicine, Charlottesville, VA.)

slight granularity on Papanicolaou stain (see Figure 7-49) and more accentuated granularity on Romanowsky stain (see Figure 7-47). The cytoplasmic granules are even more readily identified with periodic acid–Schiff (PAS) with diastase (Figure 7-52). Reports of the cytologic features of these tumors are rare [65, 68–72].

Cytology of Acinar Cell Carcinoma

- Richly cellular smears
- Large and small clusters, single cells, stripped nuclei
- Uniform cells resembling normal acinar cells
- Round to oval, central, or eccentric euchromatic nuclei with smooth nuclear contours and prominent nucleoli
- Scant to moderate cytoplasm with granularity best seen on Romanowsky stain
- PAS-positive, diastase-resistant granules
- Zymogen granules on electron microscopy

The cytoplasmic granularity is secondary to zymogen granules, which are the target of most immunocytochemical stains that aid in the identification of these tumors. All tumors are usually positive for at least one enzyme marker, but very few stain for all of them or even the same ones [56]. The immunophenotype of these tumors is outlined in Table 7-3. The most reliably present enzyme by immunocytochemistry is trypsin, and amylase is rarely detected [55, 56, 68].

The ultrastructural features of ACC are remarkably similar to normal acinar cells. The zymogen granules are in the range of 125–1,000 nm, are apically located, and

may be scanty in solid tumors [56]. These granules are generally round and homogeneous, but other studies have detected a second population of abnormal granules containing filaments that appear to be a distinguishing feature of ACC at the electron-microscopic level [56, 73]. Other ultrastructural features include tight junctions, desmosomes, short microvilli, thin basement membranes, abundant rough endoplasmic reticulin, well-formed Golgi cells, minimal to moderate amounts of glycogen, and polarized organelles (i.e., basal nuclei) [56]. Polarization is less pronounced in solid tumors [56].

Treatment of choice is surgical resection, which is correlated with slightly improved survival [56]. Other factors associated with decreased survival appear to include age at presentation (older than 60 years old), tumor size (>10 cm), tumor in the pancreatic head, and the presence of metastases at presentation, with only the first two factors being statistically significant [56].

The differential diagnosis most often includes benign pancreatic acini, pancreatic endocrine tumor (PET), solid pseudopapillary tumor (SPPT), and pancreatoblastoma (PBL). The distinguishing features of these tumors are outlined in Table 7-4.

PANCREATOBLASTOMA

PBL is an extremely rare primary pancreatic malignancy occurring almost exclusively in young children in the first decade of life [74, 75]. Only rare cases in adults have been reported [76, 77]. The male-to-female ratio is 2:1 [78], and there is a disproportionate number of cases in patients of Asian descent [74, 78]. The tumor may be

TABLE 7-3. Immunophenotype of Acinar Cell Carcinoma

Stain	Results
Trypsin	+
Chymotrypsin	–/+
Lipase	
21	–/+
105	+/–
Amylase	=/+
Keratin	+/–
Carcinoembryonic antigen	≡/+
Alpha-fetoprotein	≡/+ (focal)
Epithelial membrane antigen	≡/+ (focal)
Alpha$_1$-antitrypsin	+/–
Chromogranin	–/+
CA 19.9	–/+
B72.3	–/+
Mucin antigen MI	–

+ indicates virtually all positive; – indicates virtually all negative; –/+ indicates more tumors negative; +/– indicates more tumors positive; ≡/+ indicates most tumors negative; =/+ indicates many tumors negative.

Sources: Adapted from DS Klimstra, CS Heffess, JE Oertel, et al. Acinar cell carcinoma of the pancreas. A clinicopathologic study of 28 cases. Am J Surg Pathol 1992;16:815; and A Hoorens, F Gebhard, K Fraft, et al. Pancreatoblastoma in an adult: its separation from acinar cell carcinoma. Virchows Arch [A] 1994;424:485.

TABLE 7-4. Distinguishing Cytologic Features in the Differential Diagnosis of Acinar Cell Carcinoma

Tumor	Distinguishing Cytologic Features
ACC	Proliferation of bland-appearing acini in loosely cohesive large and small groups; epithelial naked nuclei
	PASD + cytoplasmic granules
	Trypsin and/or chymotrypsin +; amylase –
	Zymogen granules on EM
Benign acini	Mixture of acini and ductal elements
	Acini in small, grapelike clusters
PET	Small clusters with rosette formation but predominantly dyshesive cells
	Smaller cells with scant cytoplasm, which is often eccentric (plasmacytoid appearance); neuroendocrine, salt-and-pepper chromatin
	Trypsin –; chromogranin +
	Neurosecretory granules on EM
SPPT	Occurs primarily in young women
	Cytoplasmic hyaline globules, PASD +
	Branching papillary clusters with fibrovascular cores and myxoid stroma
	Vimentin, A1AT, NSE +; trypsin –
	No microvilli on EM
PBL	Two-cell populations instead of one; primitive epithelial cells and stromal cells
	± Squamoid cells

ACC = acinar cell carcinoma; EM = electron microscopy; PET = pancreatic endocrine tumor; SPPT = solid pseudopapillary tumor; PASD = periodic acid–Schiff with diastase; A1AT = alpha$_1$-antitrypsin; PBL = pancreatoblastoma.

congenital and has been reported in association with the Beckwith-Wiedemann syndrome [79–81]. Most patients, however, present with nonspecific symptoms referable to an upper abdominal mass without clear connections to a pancreatic origin. Jaundice is uncommon [78]. Radiographic studies generally illustrate a sharply defined, round to lobulated, heterogeneous mass that may be cystic and calcified [82–85].

Patients frequently have an elevated serum alphafetoprotein level, a feature that has been used clinically as a marker for tumor recurrence [86].

PBL is a highly aggressive tumor, with frequent local invasion, recurrence, and metastases. The mean survival is approximately 17 months [74]. It is rare for patients with metastatic disease to survive [74]. Despite this poor prognosis, it is a potentially curable disease if detected early and completely excised.

Grossly, PBLs are bulky, round to oval, lobulated masses that appear at least partially encapsulated and display a heterogeneous cut surface with occasional foci of hemorrhage, necrosis, and rarely grossly appreciable cysts (Figure 7-53) [74, 78, 86–89].

Histologically, these tumors are characterized by an organoid, tubuloacinar, or trabecular epithelial proliferation. They are separated by fibrovascular septae and speckled with a distinctive and ubiquitous unencapsulated globular aggregate of squamoid cells with a conspicuous peripheral-to-central gradient of maturation known as a squamoid corpuscle (Figures 7-54 and 7-55) [74, 78].

Cytologic descriptions of this tumor are rare [88]. FNAB smears demonstrate a highly cellular, predominantly dissociated smear pattern (Figures 7-56 and 7-57) composed largely of primitive, round to

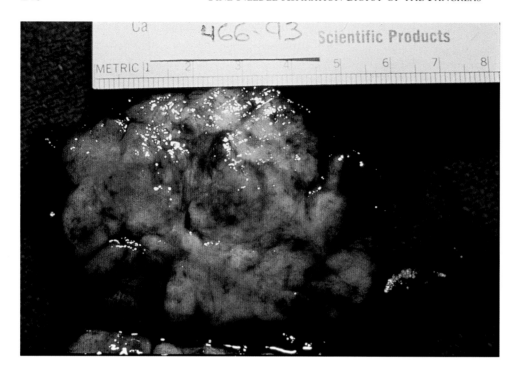

FIGURE 7-53. Pancreato-blastoma. Grossly, these tumors are bulky and lobulated and may demonstrate a variegated, focally hemorrhagic cut surface. (Courtesy of Dr. Celeste Powers, State University of New York Health Science Center, Syracuse, NY.)

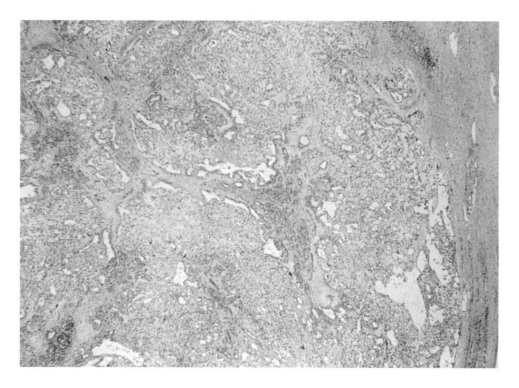

FIGURE 7-54. Pancreato-blastoma. The histomorphology of this tumor is characterized by a tubuloacinar to trabecular epithelial proliferation separated by fibrovascular septae (Hematoxylin and Eosin, 10×). (Courtesy of Dr. Celeste Powers, State University of New York Health Science Center, Syracuse, NY.)

FIGURE 7-55. Pancreato-blastoma. The distinctive feature on histomorphology is the presence of the squamoid corpuscle (Hematoxylin and Eosin, 25×). (Courtesy of Dr. Antonio Perez-Atayde, Children's Hospital, Boston.)

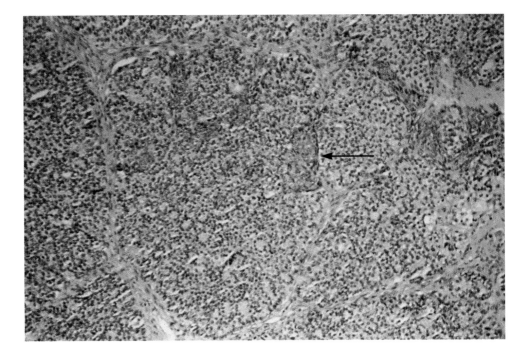

FIGURE 7-56. Pancreato-blastoma. Aspirate smears demonstrate a predominantly dissociated but cellular smear pattern (Papanicolaou, 25×). (Courtesy of Dr. Celeste Powers, State University of New York Health Science Center, Syracuse, NY.)

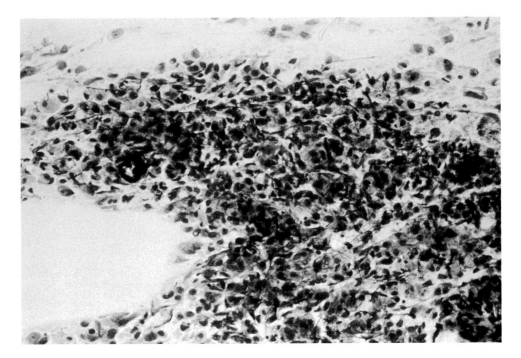

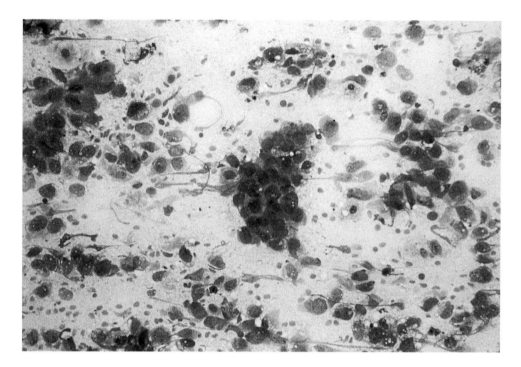

FIGURE 7-57. Pancreato-blastoma. Within the highly dissociated smear pattern, occasional cell clusters can be seen (Romanowsky, 25×). (Courtesy of Dr. Celeste Powers, State University of New York Health Science Center, Syracuse, NY.)

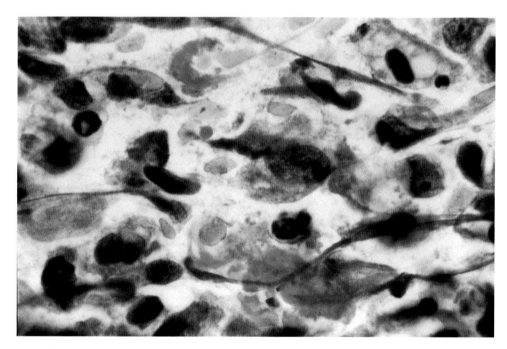

FIGURE 7-58. Pancreato-blastoma. The primitive epithelial cells show variable degrees of atypia, with central to eccentric nuclei; coarse, evenly distributed chromatin; occasional nucleoli; and delicate, finely granular cytoplasm (Papanicolaou, 25×). (Courtesy of Dr. Celeste Powers, State University of New York Health Science Center at Syracuse College of Medicine, Syracuse, NY.)

oval, and occasionally triangular epithelial cells with central to eccentric nuclei, evenly distributed coarse chromatin, occasional nucleoli, and delicate, finely granular cytoplasm (Figures 7-58 and 7-59). Mesenchymal stromal fragments with traversing capillaries, dense, acellular stromal fragments, and necrotic debris have also been described [88]. The identification of squamous corpuscles has not been described on smears and may be better appreciated on cell block preparations (Figure 7-60).

Cytology of Pancreatoblastoma

- Highly cellular smears
- Single cells, some clusters
- Primitive, blastema-type epithelial cells
- Eccentric nuclei in some cells
- Coarse, evenly distributed chromatin
- Delicate cytoplasm
- Stromal fragments
- ± Squamous cells

FIGURE 7-59. Pancreato-blastoma. The epithelial cells on Romanowsky stain demonstrate the undifferentiated, premature nature of the cells with delicate, finely granular cytoplasm (Romanowsky, 50×). (Courtesy of Dr. Celeste Powers, State University of New York Health Science Center, Syracuse, NY.)

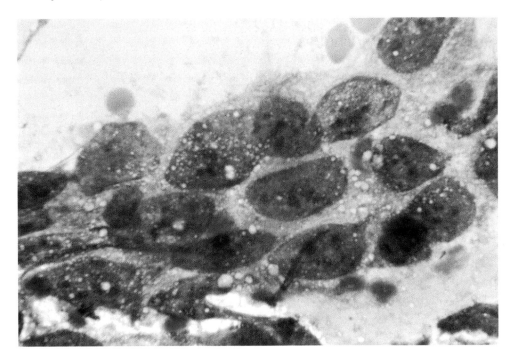

FIGURE 7-60. Pancreato-blastoma. A cell block preparation demonstrates a small cluster of squamoid-appearing cells representing a portion of a squamoid corpuscle (Hematoxylin and Eosin, 40×). (Courtesy of Dr. Celeste Powers, State University of New York Health Science Center, Syracuse, NY.)

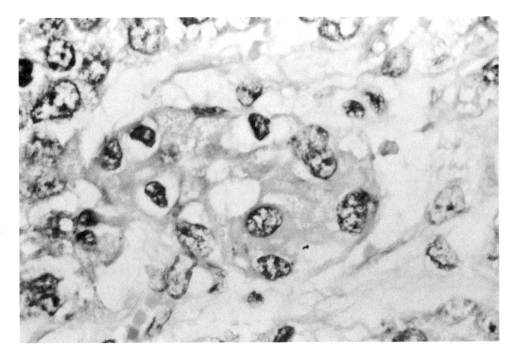

The histogenesis of PBL appears to be one of pancreatic blastema. Evidence has demonstrated differentiation in the direction of all three major cell types: acinar, endocrine, and ductal [74]. Some cells may exhibit amphocrine features as well [90]. Others have favored a ductal origin [91], acinar origin [75, 87], or a dual acinar and neuroendocrine origin [90] based on immunohistochemical or electron-microscopic findings. Acinar differentiation is the most consistently present line of differentiation [74]. As such, the most helpful immunoperoxidase stains include trypsin, chymotrypsin, and lipase. This corresponds to the demonstration of zymogen granules on electron microscopy in these cells [75]. Endocrine differentiation, albeit frequently only focal, is identifiable in more than 50% of cases with positivity to chromogranin, synaptophysin, and neuron-specific enolase (NSE) [74]. Tumor cells have also been shown to be positive for high- and low-molecular-weight cytokeratin and carcinoembryonic antigen (CEA; cytoplasmic and membranous) [88].

The differential diagnosis of PBL largely includes other pancreatic neoplasms (see Table 7-4). The defining microscopic feature of PBL is the squamoid corpuscle, which is a tremendous aid in making this diagnosis.

Ductal adenocarcinoma is extremely rare in children and is characterized by mucin-producing glands, marked nuclear pleomorphism, and desmoplastic stroma, the features of which are not associated with PBL.

ACC is probably the most difficult tumor to distinguish from PBL due to the constant finding of acinar differentiation [74]. Although these tumors are more common at opposite extremes of age (PBL in children and ACC in adults), they have been reported in all ages. ACC is differentiated by a single dominant population of acinar cells with rare endocrine elements and the lack of cellular stroma and squamoid corpuscles. The immunohistochemical profiles may overlap in some cases, but ACC generally stains more intensely and diffusely than PBL for pancreatic enzymes and much more focally than PBL for endocrine markers and CEA [56, 74].

SPPT is a clinically and microscopically distinct entity that should not be confused with PBL (see discussion of SPPT in Chapter 6).

Pancreatic endocrine tumors (PETs) are rare in the first decade of life and are distinguished from PBL by their lack of cellular stroma and squamoid corpuscles. Endocrine markers are also more diffuse than focal.

PANCREATIC ENDOCRINE TUMORS

Panoreatic endocrine tumors (PETs) are rare. Clinically silent tumors have been found in 0.4–1.6% of pancreases in unselected autopsy studies [92]. They comprise 0.5–4.0% of all primary pancreatic neoplasms [93, 94].

PETs have been theorized to develop from ductular stem cells, but this hypothesis remains unproved [96]. PETs derive from cells of the diffuse neuroendocrine-endocrine system. As such, these tumors show markers of neuroendocrine differentiation, including NSE, synaptophysin, chromogranin A and C, Leu 7, and the production of regulatory peptides, hormones, and amines. Electron microscopy shows electron-dense, membrane-bound granules [95].

Most PETs occur in adults, although they have been reported in children [96]. Functional neoplasms produce a number of hormonal syndromes, classified according to the primary hormone being produced [95, 96]. However, production of multiple hormones and the presence of more than one cell type have been shown [97–100]. Functioning types account for 60–85% of all PETs [95]. PETs that do not produce a clinically recognized syndrome or that lack elevated hormone levels are referred to as nonfunctioning.

Insulinomas are the most frequently occurring functional PET; 70–99% are benign [95]. Most are solitary, but patients with multiple endocrine neoplasia type I (MEN I) may have multiple insulinomas. Whipple's triad is characteristic of this tumor and consists of (1) symptoms of hypoglycemia, such as fatigue, convulsions, weakness, mental confusion; (2) low fasting blood glucose levels; and (3) relief of symptoms by the administration of glucose [96, 101]. Immunohistochemical studies show insulin in almost all tumors, and 50% are multihormonal [95]. Typical beta granules are seen on electron microscopy [95].

Glucagonomas are usually large and solitary; 60% are malignant [95]. Most occur in adults. Unlike most other PETs, glucagonoma shows a female predilection. Immunohistochemistry shows weak staining of tumor cells for glucagon and immunoreactivity to proglucagon hormones [95]. Electron microscopy shows type A granules in nonfunctioning tumors and atypical granules in functioning tumors. The glucagonoma syndrome is characterized by necrolytic migratory erythema, mild glucose intolerance, normocytic anemia, weight loss, and deep vein thrombosis [96].

Gastrinomas occur predominantly in adults and in males. Excessive gastrin secretion produces the Zollinger-Ellison syndrome. The sporadic forms tend to be larger, and 60% are malignant [95]. Those associated with MEN I are multicentric and less likely to be malignant (25–30%) [95]. Immunohistochemical studies demonstrate gastrin in most cells, and 50% are multihormonal. The electron-microscopic findings are not specific [95].

Vasoactive intestinal polypeptide–producing tumors (VIPomas) produce the Verner-Morrison syndrome, also known as the WDHA syndrome (WDHA stands for watery diarrhea, hypokalemia, and achlorhydria). Approximately 80% of these tumors are malignant [95]. VIPomas show a female predilection just as glucagonomas. Most are solitary, large tumors. VIPomas frequently contain pancreatic polypeptide (PP)–producing cells, in addition to cells secreting vasoactive intestinal polypeptide. Electron microscopy shows small granules [95].

The clinical findings associated with somatostatinoma include diabetes mellitus, cholecystolithiasis, steatorrhea, indigestion, hypochlorhydria, and anemia. Most occur in the duodenum at the site of the ampulla of Vater or close to it [96]. They are also associated with von Recklinghausen's disease or pheochromocytoma [95]. Pancreatic polypeptide-producing tumors (PPomas) do not have a well-defined clinical syndrome. Tumors that produce only pancreatic polypeptide are rare, and these types of cells are usually a component of other tumors [101]. Other rare types of PET include neurotensinomas and calcitoninomas [95].

Multihormonality is a frequent finding in tumors associated with MEN I. PPomas are the most frequent type, followed by glucagonomas and insulinomas. Tumors occurring in MEN I are usually benign [95].

FIGURE 7-61. Pancreatic endocrine tumor. Gross photograph of resection specimen showing well-circumscribed, pink, fleshy tumor mass with central, yellow necrosis.

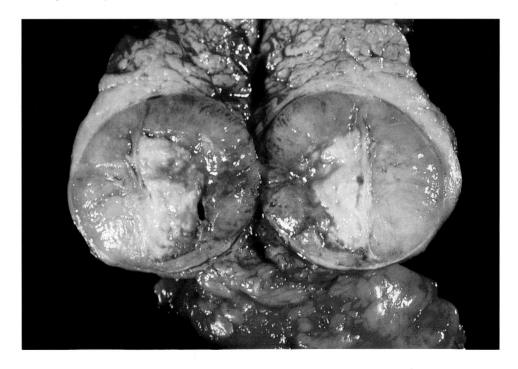

The only definitive criteria for malignancy are gross invasion of adjacent organs; metastases to regional lymph nodes, liver, and other distant sites; or blood vessel invasion, the latter being the only histologic marker of malignancy [96]. Other parameters associated with outcome include tumor size, mitotic activity, tumor necrosis, perineural invasion, type of hormone secretion, and presence or absence of hormonal syndrome [96]. These parameters can be used to grade the differentiated tumors according to their malignant potential as benign, borderline, and low-grade carcinomas [96]. In general, tumors of less than 2 cm are benign; tumors of more than 3 cm usually demonstrate malignant behavior, with exceptions; and tumors between 2 and 3 cm demonstrate an intermediate potential for malignant behavior. Vascular and perineural space invasion have been observed in more than 90% of malignant PETs associated with distant metastases [96]. Tumors with more than two to four mitoses per high-power field usually behave as low-grade carcinomas. Insulinomas are usually benign, whereas tumors that produce other types of syndromes and nonfunctional tumors have a greater chance for recurrence or metastases. A combination of parameters is needed to make an informed decision concerning a tumor's potential for malignant behavior. Poorly differentiated endocrine carcinomas with widespread tumor necrosis, a high mitotic index, and anaplasia, otherwise classified as small cell carcinoma, are all malignant and follow an aggressive course [102].

Reliable serum, immunohistochemical, and other adjunctive markers have been sought to predict behavior. One such marker, DNA ploidy, has been evaluated, but it does not predict behavior independently of other parameters [103]. Contrary to earlier reports, alpha human chorionic gonadotropin levels do not correlate with malignant behavior either [104]. Proliferative indices have been evaluated using Ki-67 and proliferating cell nuclear antigen, and both appear to distinguish benign from low-grade malignant neoplasms [96, 105]; however, their long-term applicability has yet to be determined.

Grossly, these tumors appear as well-circumscribed, fleshy, pinkish masses in the pancreas (Figure 7-61), which may be associated with central necrosis. Four histomorphologic patterns are recognized [101]: trabecular, solid, glandular, and nondescript (Figure 7-62). Histologically, the tumors are composed of uniform, cuboidal cells with central nuclei and acidophilic or amphophilic cytoplasm that varies in quantity. The nuclei are round to oval with finely stippled chromatin and occasionally small nucleoli (Figure 7-63). Pleomorphism and mitoses may be seen. Psammoma bodies have been described as a not uncommon finding [106]. The stroma is highly vascular and may contain abundant hyaline material [101]. Amyloid deposition in the stroma may be encountered, particularly in insulin-secreting tumors [101].

A clear cell variant with vacuolated cytoplasm that contains cytoplasmic lipid by electron microscopy has been reported [107]. Ferreiro et al. described an islet cell tumor with rhabdomyosarcomatous differentiation [108].

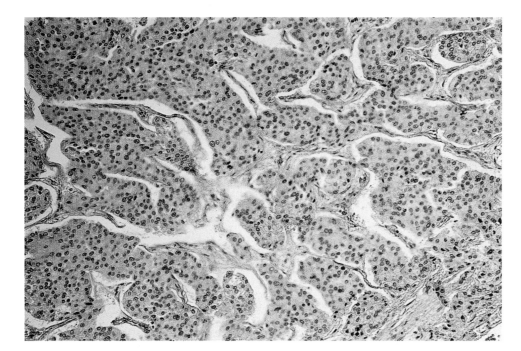

FIGURE 7-62. Pancreatic endocrine tumor. Medium-power view of histology specimen showing trabeculae of tumor cells surrounded by fibrovascular stroma (Hematoxylin and Eosin, 20×).

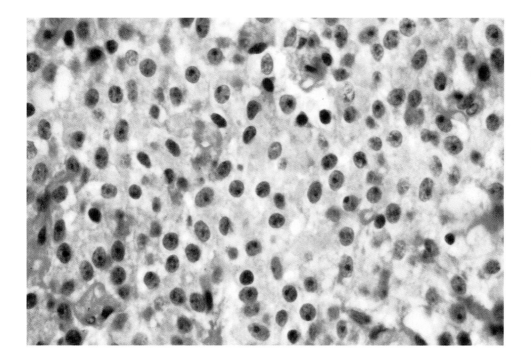

FIGURE 7-63. Pancreatic endocrine tumor. The nuclei of these tumors are typically round and uniform with a salt-and-pepper chromatin pattern and small nucleoli. The cytoplasm is eosinophilic and variable in quantity (Hematoxylin and Eosin, 40×).

FIGURE 7-64. Pancreatic endocrine tumor. Very cellular smear in which homogenous, single tumor cells are evenly dispersed on the slide (Papanicolaou, 25×).

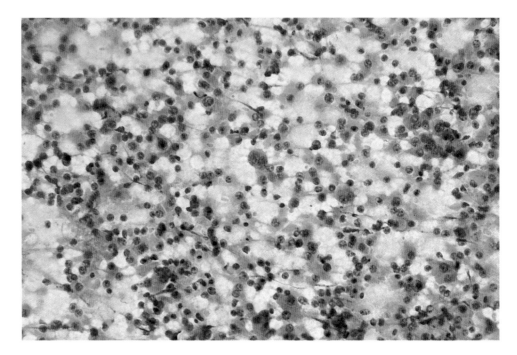

FIGURE 7-65. Pancreatic endocrine tumor. Clusters of neoplastic cells forming a rosette (Papanicolaou, 40×; ×1.6 optivar).

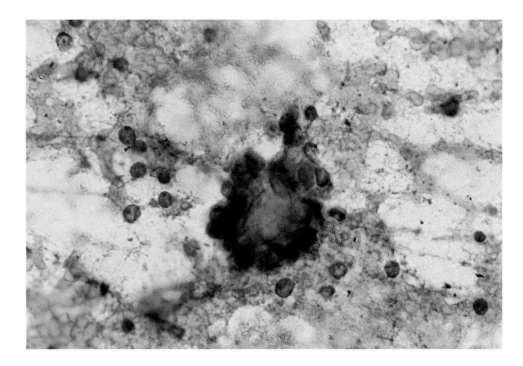

Other variants include a mucinous variant, which contained goblet cells [109], and an oncocytic variant [110].

A number of reports have described the cytologic findings of PET [111–115]. The most recent review article by Collins and Cramer [111] summarized the cytologic findings in their own study and in the literature. The FNAB smears of PET are typically very cellular and composed of a homogeneous population of dyshesive cells (Figure 7-64). In most cases, single cells predominate, but the cells may aggregate in loose groups or rosette-like structures (Figure 7-65) or form sheets with poorly defined borders (Figure 7-66). Fibrovascular stroma surrounded by loosely attached tumor cells are another feature, correlating with the vascular stroma seen on histopathology (Figures 7-67 and 7-68). The nuclei are round and uniform, with smooth nuclear membranes and a finely stip-

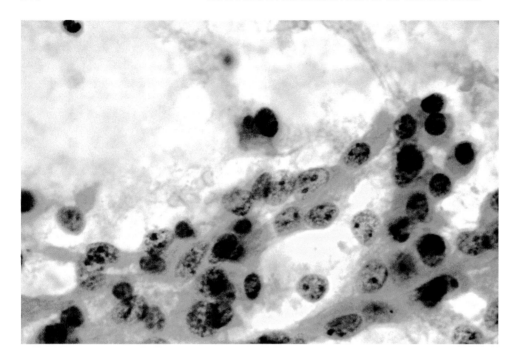

Figure 7-66. Pancreatic endocrine tumor. Group of tumor cells in a loosely cohesive fragment with ill-defined, basophilic, wispy cytoplasm (Papanicolaou, 40×; ×1.25 optivar).

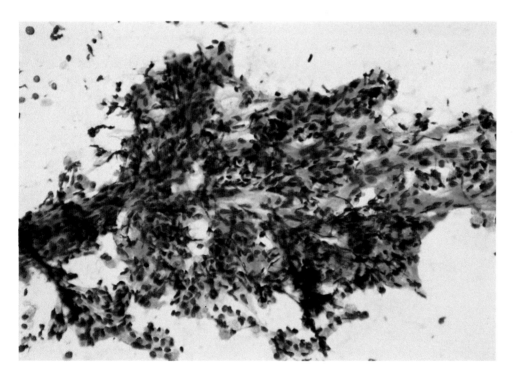

FIGURE 7-67. Pancreatic endocrine tumor. Fibrovascular stroma containing delicate endothelial channels and surrounded by neoplastic cells (Papanicolaou, 20×).

FIGURE 7-68. Pancreatic endocrine tumor, clear cell variant. Vascular stromal fragment with a few loosely attached neoplastic cells (modified Wright-Giemsa, 40×).

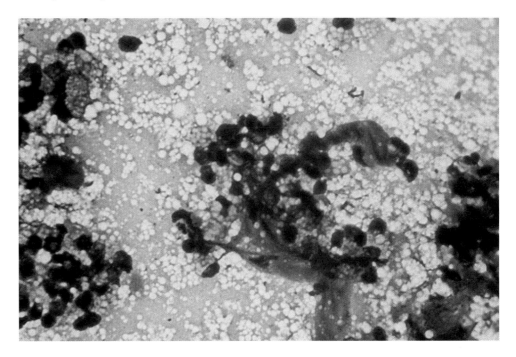

FIGURE 7-69. Pancreatic endocrine tumor. Loose clusters of tumor cells with wispy, basophilic, ill-defined cytoplasm and central round, homogenous nuclei having a finely stippled chromatin (Papanicolaou, 63×).

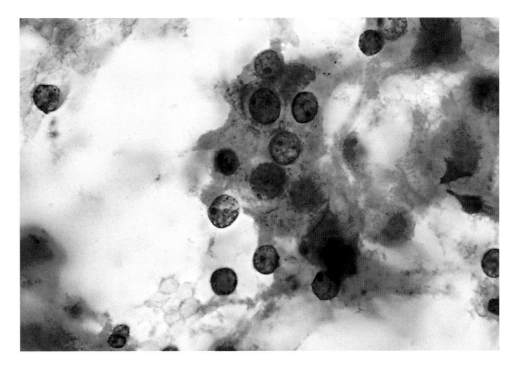

pled chromatin pattern. The cytoplasm is basophilic, wispy, and ill defined (Figure 7-69). Some cells may have abundant well-defined, dense cytoplasm and eccentrically placed nuclei, which imparts a plasmacytoid appearance to the cells (Figure 7-70). The clear cell variant has cytoplasmic vacuolization due to the presence of lipid deposition (Figure 7-71). Binucleation and multinucleation (Figure 7-72), coarse chromatin, nucleoli, and mitotic figures may be found (Figure 7-73) and do not predict the behavior of the tumor. There are no proven cytologic correlates of malignancy [111]. Immunohistochemical studies demonstrate positivity for neuroendocrine markers (Figure 7-74). Dense core granules are seen on electron microscopy (Figures 7-75 and 7-76).

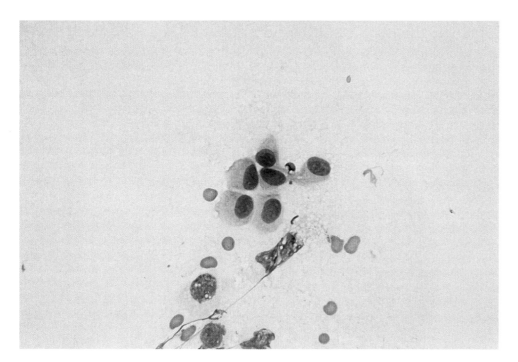

FIGURE 7-70. Pancreatic endocrine tumor. Plasmacytoid tumor cells with abundant dense, sharply defined cytoplasm and eccentric nuclei (modified Wright-Giemsa, 40×; ×1.25 optivar).

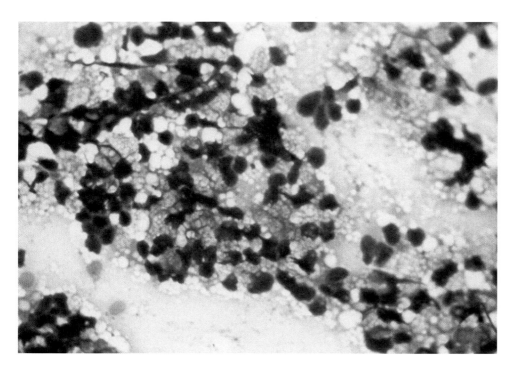

FIGURE 7-71. Pancreatic endocrine tumor, clear cell variant. The tumor cells have abundant vacuolated cytoplasm (modified Wright-Giemsa, 40×).

FIGURE 7-72. Pancreatic endocrine tumor. Tumor has abundant, dense, granular cytoplasm. The nuclei are enlarged, the chromatin is coarse and clumpy, and a multinucleated cell is seen (Papanicolaou, 100×).

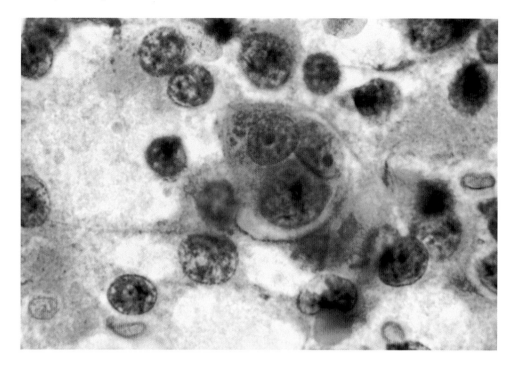

FIGURE 7-73. Pancreatic endocrine tumor. Different field from the case shown in Figure 7-72 with a mitotic figure (Papanicolaou, 100×; ×1.6 optivar).

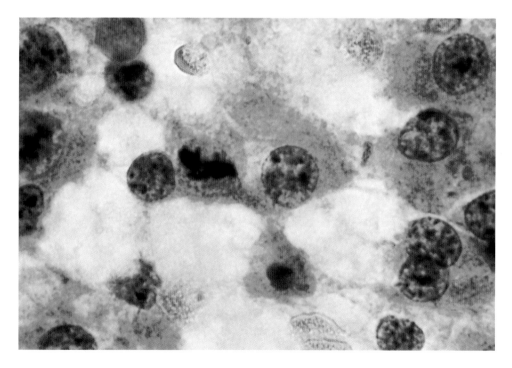

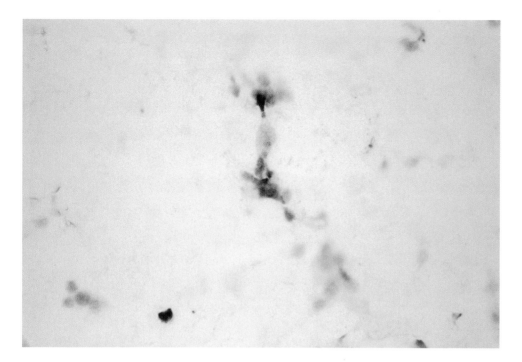

FIGURE 7-74. Pancreatic endocrine tumor. Immunohistochemical study showing positivity for chromogranin (immunoperoxidase, 40×).

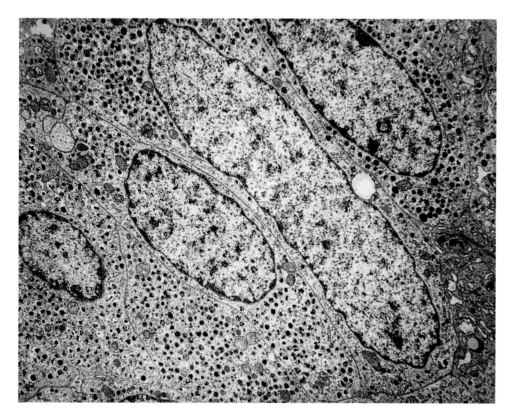

FIGURE 7-75. Pancreatic endocrine tumor. Low magnification reveals oval and elongated cells having a rich collection of cytoplasmic granules (electron microscopy, 7000×). (Courtesy of Dr. G. Richard Dickersin, Harvard Medical School, Massachusetts General Hospital, Boston).

FIGURE 7-76. Pancreatic endocrine tumor. High magnification of cytoplasmic granules from the same cytoplasm shown in Figure 7-75 reveals them to be of the dense core type, with many of the cores having the angular, crystalline structure of beta granules (electron microscopy, 22,300×). (Courtesy of Dr. G. Richard Dickersin, Harvard Medical School, Massachusetts General Hospital, Boston.)

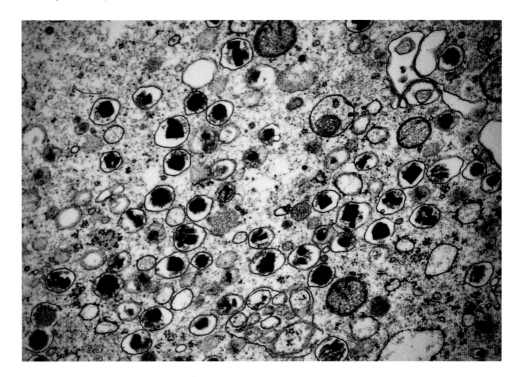

Cytomorphology of Pancreatic Endocrine Tumors

- High cellularity
- Monotonous, extremely dyshesive, cell population
- Loose groups and rosette-like structures
- Vascular stroma with attached, loose, cohesive neoplastic cells
- Round to oval, eccentrically placed nuclei with finely stippled or coarsely granular chromatin
- Basophilic, wispy, and ill-defined or dense and sharply defined cytoplasm
- Binucleation or multinucleation, mitoses, small nucleoli, and pleomorphism variably present

The differential diagnoses include the following:

- Endocrine cell proliferations, such as endocrine cell hyperplasia or nesidioblastosis
- ACC
- Neuroendocrine carcinoma or small cell carcinoma
- SPPT
- Adenocarcinoma
- Malignant lymphoma
- Other plasmacytoid neoplasms, such as plasmacytomas and malignant melanoma

Hyperplasia of pancreatic endocrine cells, as may arise in chronic pancreatitis, demonstrates groups of endocrine cells in clusters with occasional glandular formation. The cells have a filmy, ill-defined cytoplasm and round to oval, slightly hyperchromatic nuclei with small nucleoli [116] and are associated with pancreatic exocrine cells. The scant number of groups, the admixture of endocrine and exocrine cells, and the cohesiveness contrast with the cellularity and dyshesion seen in PET (Figure 7-77). Immunoperoxidase studies confirm the neuroendocrine nature of these groups (Figure 7-78) because they may resemble acinar cells.

As the hyperplasia becomes more complex and proliferative, distinguishing hyperplasia from PET becomes much more difficult, if not impossible [117].

The differential diagnosis from ACC is discussed in "Acinar Cell Carcinoma," and an approach to the differential diagnosis is described in Table 7-4.

The differential diagnosis from SPPT of the pancreas is discussed in Chapter 6, and the cytologic differential diagnosis is reiterated in Table 7-4.

Neuroendocrine carcinomas have more readily apparent necrosis and mitotic activity [118]. The nuclei may also be more hyperchromatic and fusiform.

In contrast to PET, the cells of adenocarcinoma occur in clusters more often than singly. The nuclei exhibit nuclear membrane irregularities, prominent nucleoli, and abnormalities of chromatin distribution not seen in PET [114]. The presence of cytoplasmic mucin vacuoles in adenocarcinomas differentiate them from PET [111].

The dyshesion of the neoplastic cells in PET and the scant cytoplasm may suggest malignant lymphoma [114]. However, PETs show cohesive groups, and in some areas, the cytoplasm is more abundant than it is in lymphomas. When in doubt, immunoperoxidase studies

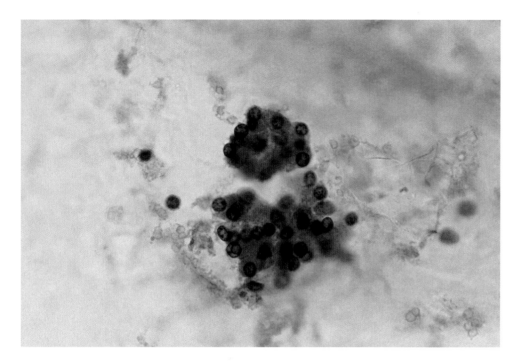

FIGURE 7-77. Islet cell hyperplasia. Islet cells in small clusters with ill-defined basophilic cytoplasm and round, uniform nuclei. These groups were few in number on the smear and were associated with pancreatic exocrine elements (Papanicolaou, 40×; ×1.6 optivar).

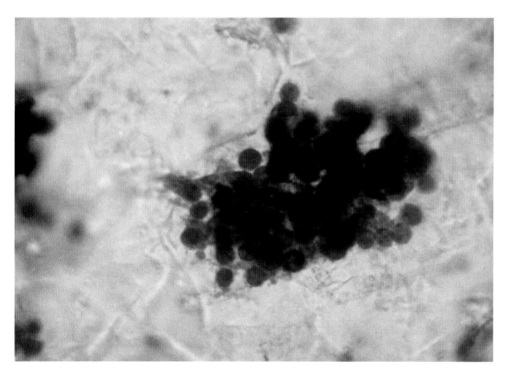

FIGURE 7-78. Islet cell hyperplasia. The cells are positive for chromogranin (immunoperoxidase, 40×).

FIGURE 7-79. Small cell carcinoma. Very cellular fine needle aspiration biopsy smear showing malignant cells occurring singly or in loose clusters and numerous crushed nuclei. A mitotic figure is seen in the cluster, and abundant background necrosis is readily apparent (Papanicolaou, 40×; ×1.6 optivar).

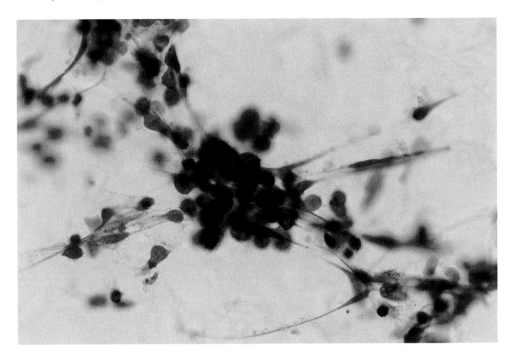

or flow cytometric immunophenotyping studies will help in the differential diagnosis.

When considering the differential diagnosis of a plasmacytoid neoplasm in an extramedullary site, endocrine neoplasms are primary on the list. However, extramedullary plasmacytomas have been reported in the pancreas [119]. Aggregates or rosette-like clusters are indicative of PET but may not be apparent in all cases. In such instances, immunohistochemical studies for keratins, chromogranin, kappa and lambda light chains, and perhaps other hormones are necessary for the differential diagnosis. Aspirates of malignant melanoma (although typically producing smears composed of single, pleomorphic cells with prominent nucleoli, intranuclear cytoplasmic inclusions, and scattered bi- or multinucleated cells) may occasionally produce a homogeneous population of plasmacytoid cells. Immunoperoxidase studies for S-100 and HMB-45 are necessary for this distinction [120].

MIXED DUCTAL-ENDOCRINE NEOPLASM

Mixed ductal-endocrine neoplasm is rare, accounting for less than 1% of all pancreatic exocrine neoplasms [1]. It consists of a mixture of ductal and endocrine cells in which 30% or more of the neoplasm is composed of endocrine cells [1, 29].

Cells with features of both endocrine and ductal differentiation have been referred to as amphicrine cells [121].

SMALL CELL CARCINOMA

Small cell carcinomas, which are considered to be poorly differentiated endocrine carcinomas, account for 1% of all pancreatic malignancies and 2–3% of all PETs [96]. These highly malignant neoplasms are similar to pulmonary and extrapulmonary, small to intermediate cell carcinomas; patients present with symptoms of advanced malignant disease, including weight loss, jaundice, and metastases [96]. Paraneoplastic syndromes are rare in pancreatic tumors: Only one adrenocorticotropin hormone (ACTH)–producing tumor and a tumor associated with hypercalcemia have been reported [122, 123]. The gross and histopathologic features are similar to small cell carcinoma of the lung. FNAB smears are very cellular and are characterized by malignant cells singly or in loose clusters that smear when spread. Mitoses are typically numerous, and background, coagulative tumor–type necrosis is readily apparent (Figure 7-79). The nuclei are hyperchromatic and oval to fusiform (Figure 7-80). Nuclear molding is a prominent feature (Figure 7-81).

Cytology of Small Cell Carcinoma

- Very cellular
- Polygonal or fusiform, hyperchromatic nuclei
- Nuclear molding
- Scant cytoplasm
- Abundant necrosis and mitoses

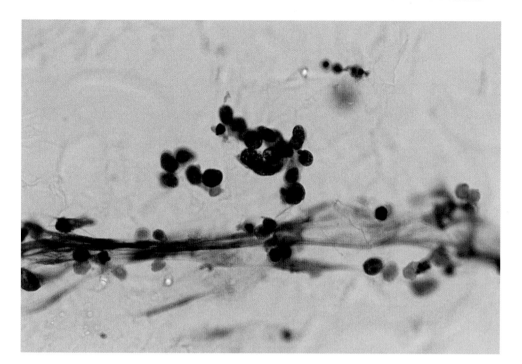

FIGURE 7-80. Small cell carcinoma. The nuclei are oval to fusiform and hyperchromatic (Papanicolaou, 40×; ×1.6 optivar).

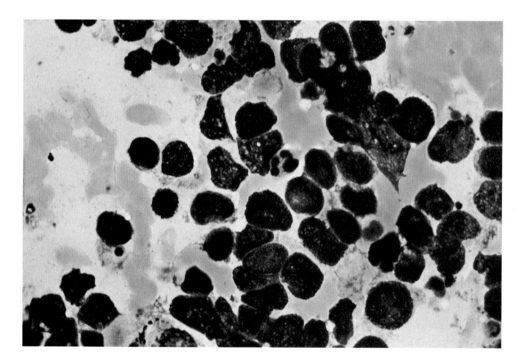

FIGURE 7-81. Small cell carcinoma. Oval to fusiform nuclei with extensive nuclear molding (modified Wright-Giemsa, 100×). (Courtesy of Dr. William J. Frable, Virginia Commonwealth University/Medical College of Virginia School of Medicine, Richmond, VA.)

REFERENCES

1. Klöppel G, Solcia E, Longnecker DS, et al. Histological Typing of Tumours of the Exocrine Pancreas (2nd ed). Berlin: Springer-Verlag, 1996.

2. Warshaw AL, Fernández-Del Castillo C. Pancreatic carcinoma. N Engl J Med 1992;326:455.

3. Murr MM, Sarr MG, Oishi AJ, et al. Pancreatic cancer. CA Cancer J Clin 1994;44:304.

4. Trede M, Schwall G, Saeger HD. Survival after pancreatoduodenectomy. Ann Surg 1990;211:447.

5. Cameron JL, Crist DW, Sitzmann JV, et al. Factors influencing survival after pancreaticoduodenectomy for pancreatic cancer. Am J Surg 1991;161:120.

6. Compton CC, Henson DE. for Members of the Cancer Committee, College of American Pathologists. Protocol for the examination of specimens removed from patients with carcinoma of the exocrine pancreas. A basis for checklists. Arch Pathol Lab Med 1997;121:1129.

7. Ettinghausen SE, Schwartzentruber DJ, Sindelar WF. Evolving strategies for the treatment of adenocarcinoma of the pancreas. A review. J Clin Gastroenterol 1995;21:48.

8. Ekberg O, Bergenfeldt M, Aspelin P, et al. Reliability of ultrasound-guided fine-needle biopsy of pancreatic masses. Acta Radiol 1988;29:535.

9. Pinto MM, Avila NA, Criscuolo EM. Fine needle aspiration of the pancreas. A five-year experience. Acta Cytol 1988;32:39.

10. Hall-Craggs MA, Lees WR. Fine-needle aspiration biopsy: pancreatic and biliary tumors. AJR Am J Roentgenol 1986;147:399.

11. Bret PM, Nicolet V, Labadie M. Percutaneous fine-needle aspiration biopsy of the pancreas. Diagn Cytopathol 1986;2:221.

12. Fekete PS, Nunez C, Pitlik DA. Fine-needle aspiration biopsy of the pancreas: a study of 61 cases. Diagn Cytopathol 1986;2:301.

13. Phillips VM, Hersh T, Erwin BC, et al. Percutaneous biopsy of pancreatic masses. J Clin Gastroenterol 1985;7:506.

14. Alpern GA, Dekker A. Fine needle aspiration cytology of the pancreas. An analysis of its use in 52 patients. Acta Cytol 1985;29:873.

15. An-Foraker SH, Fong-Mui KK. Cytodiagnosis of lesions of the pancreas and related areas. Acta Cytol 1982;26:814.

16. Kolins MD, Bernacki EG Jr, Schwab R. Diagnosis of pancreatic lesions by percutaneous aspiration biopsy. Acta Cytol 1981;25:675.

17. Athlin L, Blind PJ, Angstrom T. Fine-needle aspiration biopsy of pancreatic masses. Acta Chir Scand 1990;156:91.

18. Kim K, Booth R, Myles J. Transcutaneous fine-needle aspiration biopsy of pancreatic cancer. Int J Pancreatol 1990;7:61.

19. Parsons LJ, Palmer CH. How accurate is fine-needle biopsy in malignant neoplasia of the pancreas? Arch Surg 1989;124:681.

20. Robins DB, Katz RL, Evans DB, et al. Fine needle aspiration of the pancreas. In quest of accuracy. Acta Cytol 1995;39:1.

21. Stiles TE, Katz RL, Evans D, et al. Cytologic nuclear grading of fine needle aspirations of pancreatic adenocarcinoma as a clinicocytopathologic prognostic predictor. Mod Pathol 1997;10:39A.

22. Yamaguchi K, Enjoji M. Adenosquamous carcinoma of the pancreas: a clinicopathologic study. J Surg Oncol 1991;47:109.

23. Cihak RW, Kawashima T, Steer A. Adenoacanthoma (adenosquamous carcinoma) of the pancreas. Cancer 1972;29:1133.

24. Smit W, Mathy JP, Donaldson E. Pancreatic cytology and adenosquamous carcinoma of the pancreas. Pathology 1993;25:420.

25. Frias-Hidvegi D. Adenocarcinoma of the Pancreas. In D Frias-Hidvegi (ed), Guides to Clinical Aspiration Biopsy: Liver and Pancreas. Tokyo: Igaku-Shoin, 1988;255.

26. Wilczynski SP, Valente PT, Atkinson BF. Cytodiagnosis of adenosquamous carcinoma of the pancreas. Use of intraoperative fine needle aspiration. Acta Cytol 1984;28:733.

27. Chen J, Baithun SI, Ramsay MA. Histogenesis of pancreatic carcinomas: a study based on 248 cases. J Pathol 1985;146:65.

28. Cubilla AL, Fitzgerald PJ. Classification of pancreatic cancer (nonendocrine). Mayo Clin Proc 1979;54:449.

29. Solcia E, Capella C, Klöppel G. Tumors of the Exocrine Pancreas. In E Solcia, C Capella, G Klöppel (eds), Atlas of Tumor Pathology: Tumors of the Pancreas (3rd ed). Washington, DC: Armed Forces Institute of Pathology, 1997;31.

30. Huntrakoon M. Oncocytic carcinoma of the pancreas. Cancer 1983;51:332.

31. Nozawa Y, Abe M, Sakuma H, et al. A case of pancreatic oncocytic tumor. Acta Pathol Jpn 1990; 40:367.

32. Kanai N, Nagaki S, Tanaka T. Clear cell carcinoma of the pancreas. Acta Pathol Jpn 1987;37:1521.

33. Morinaga S, Tsumuraya M, Nakajima T, et al. Ciliated-cell adenocarcinoma of the pancreas. Acta Pathol Jpn 1986;36:1905.

34. Walts AE. Osteoclast-type giant-cell tumor of the pancreas. Acta Cytol 1983;27:500.

35. Manci EA, Gardner LL, Pollock WJ, et al. Osteoclastic giant cell tumor of the pancreas. Aspiration cytology, light microscopy, and ultrastructure with review of the literature. Diagn Cytopathol 1985;1:105.

36. Silverman JF, Finley JL, MacDonald KGJ. Fine-needle aspiration cytology of osteoclastic giant-cell tumor of the pancreas. Diagn Cytopathol 1990;6:336.

37. Rosai J. Carcinoma of pancreas simulating giant cell tumor of bone. Electron-microscopic evidence of its acinar cell origin. Cancer 1968;22:333.

38. Fischer HP, Altmannsberger M, Kracht J. Osteoclast-type giant cell tumour of the pancreas [review]. Virchows Arch [A] 1988;412:247.

39. Freund U. Pleomorphic giant cell tumor of the pancreas. A case report. Isr J Med Sci 1973;9:84.

40. Alguacil-Garcia A, Weiland LH. The histologic spectrum, prognosis, and histogenesis of the sarcomatoid carcinoma of the pancreas. Cancer 1977; 39:1181.

41. Trepeta RW, Mathur B, Lagin S, et al. Giant cell tumor ("osteoclastoma") of the pancreas: a tumor of epithelial origin. Cancer 1981;48:2022.

42. Cubilla AL, Fitzgerald PJ. Cancer of the pancreas (nonendocrine): a suggested morphologic classification. Semin Oncol 1979;6:285.

43. Shamblin WR, Priestly JT, Sprague RG, et al. Total pancreatectomy for pleomorphic carcinoma: a five year cure. Arch Surg 1966;92:315.

44. Lewandrowski KB, Weston L, Dickersin GR, et al. Giant cell tumor of the pancreas of mixed osteoclastic and pleomorphic cell type: evidence for a histogenetic relationship and mesenchymal differentiation. Hum Pathol 1990;21:1184.

45. Robinson L, Damjenov I, Brezina P. Multinucleated giant cell neoplasm of pancreas: light and electron microscopy features. Arch Pathol Lab Med 1977;101:590.

46. Berendt RC, Shnitka TK, Wiens E, et al. The osteoclast-type giant cell tumor of the pancreas. Arch Pathol Lab Med 1987;111:43.

47. Sommers SC, Meissner WA. Unusual carcinomas of the pancreas. Arch Pathol 1954;58:101.

48. Wolfman NT, Karstaedt N, Kawamoto EH. Pleomorphic carcinoma of the pancreas: computed-tomographic, sonographic, and pathologic findings. Radiology 1985;154:329.

49. Reyes CV, Crain S, Wang T. Pleomorphic giant cell carcinoma of the pancreas: a review of nine cases. J Surg Oncol 1980;15:345.

50. Pinto MM, Monteiro NL, Tizol DM. Fine needle aspiration of pleomorphic giant-cell carcinoma of the pancreas. Case report with ultrastructural observations. Acta Cytol 1986;30:430.

51. Silverman JF, Finley JL, Berns L, et al. Significance of giant cells in fine-needle aspiration biopsies of benign and malignant lesions of the pancreas. Diagn Cytopathol 1989;5:388.

52. Frable WJ. Thin Needle Aspiration Biopsy. Philadelphia: Saunders, 1983.

53. Chen J, Baithun SI. Morphological study of 391 cases of exocrine pancreatic tumours with special reference to the classification of exocrine pancreatic carcinoma. J Pathol 1985;146:17.

54. Cubilla AL, Fitzgerald PJ. Morphological patterns of primary nonendocrine human pancreas carcinoma. Cancer Res 1975;35:2234.

55. Morohoshi T, Held G, Kloppel G. Pancreatic tumors and their histological classification: a study based on 167 autopsy and 97 surgical cases. Histopathology 1983;7:645.

56. Klimstra DS, Heffess CS, Oertel JE, et al. Acinar cell carcinoma of the pancreas. A clinicopathologic study of 28 cases. Am J Surg Pathol 1992;16:815.

57. Baylor SM, Berg JW. Cross-classification and survival characteristics of 5000 cases of cancer of the pancreas. J Surg Oncol 1973;5:335.

58. Mah PT, Loo DC, Tock EPC. Pancreatic acinar cell carcinoma in childhood. Am J Dis Child 1990; 128:101.

59. Osborne BM, Culbert SJ, Cangir A, et al. Acinar cell carcinoma of the pancreas in a 9-year-old child: case report with electron microscopic observations. South Med J 1977;70:370.

60. Alcantara EN. Functioning acinar cell carcinoma of the pancreas. Can Med Assoc J 1962;87:970.

61. Auger C. Acinous cell carcinoma of the pancreas with extensive fat necrosis. Arch Pathol 1947; 43:400.

62. Belsky H, Cornell NW. Disseminated focal fat necrosis following radical pancreatoduodenectomy for acinous carcinoma of head of pancreas. Ann Surg 1955;141:556.

63. Burns WA, Matthews MJ, Hamosh M, et al. Lipase-secreting acinar cell carcinoma of the pancreas with polyarthropathy. Cancer 1974;33:1002.

64. Radin DR, Colletti PM, Forrester DM, et al. Pancreatic acinar cell carcinoma with subcutaneous and intraosseous fat necrosis. Radiology 1986;158:67.

65. Ishihara A, Sanda T, Takanari H, et al. Elastase-1-secreting acinar cell carcinoma of the pancreas. A cytologic, electron microscopic and histochemical study. Acta Cytol 1989;33:157.

66. Stamm B, Burger H, Hollinger A. Acinar cell cystadenocarcinoma of the pancreas. Cancer 1987; 60:2542.

67. Cantrell BB, Cubilla AL, Erlandson RA, et al. Acinar cell cystadenocarcinoma of human pancreas. Cancer 1981;47:410.

68. Labate AM, Klimstra DL, Zakowski MF. Comparative cytologic features of pancreatic acinar cell carcinoma and islet cell tumor. Diagn Cytopathol 1997;16:112.

69. Geisinger KR, Silverman JF. Fine-Needle Aspiration Cytology of Uncommon Primary Pancreatic Neoplasms: A Personal Experience and Review of the Literature. In WA Schmidt (ed), Cytopathology Annual. Baltimore: Williams & Wilkins, 1992;23.

70. Villanueva RR, Nguyen-Ho P, Nguyen GK. Needle aspiration cytology of acinar-cell carcinoma of the pancreas: report of a case with diagnostic pitfalls and

unusual ultrastructural findings. Diagn Cytopathol 1994;10:362.

71. Samuel LH, Frierson HJ. Fine needle aspiration cytology of acinar cell carcinoma of the pancreas: a report of two cases. Acta Cytol 1996;40:585.

72. Silverman JF, Geisinger KR. Ancillary studies in FNA of liver and pancreas. Diagn Cytopathol 1995;13:396.

73. Tucker JA, Shelburne JD, Benning TL, et al. Filamentous inclusions in acinar cell carcinoma of the pancreas. Ultrastruct Pathol 1994;18:279.

74. Klimstra DS, Wenig BM, Adair CF, et al. Pancreatoblastoma. A clinicopathologic study and review of the literature [review]. Am J Surg Pathol 1995;19:1371.

75. Morohoshi T, Kanda M, Horie A, et al. Immunocytochemical markers of uncommon pancreatic tumors. Acinar cell carcinoma, pancreatoblastoma, and solid cystic (papillary-cystic) tumor. Cancer 1987;59:739.

76. Hoorens A, Gebhard F, Fraft K, et al. Pancreatoblastoma in an adult: its separation from acinar cell carcinoma. Virchows Arch [A] 1994;424:485.

77. Palosaari D, Clayton F, Seaman J. Pancreatoblastoma in an adult. Arch Pathol Lab Med 1986; 110:1494.

78. Kissane JM. Pancreatoblastoma and solid and cystic papillary tumor: two tumors related to pancreatic ontogeny. Semin Diagn Pathol 1994;11:152.

79. Drut R, Jones MC. Congenital pancreatoblastoma in Beckwith-Wiedemann syndrome: an emerging association. Pediatr Pathol Lab Med 1988;8:331.

80. Koh THHG, Cooper JE, Newman CL, et al. Pancreatoblastoma in a neonate with Wiedemann-Beckwith syndrome. Eur J Pediatr 1986;145:435.

81. Potts SR, Brown S, O'Hara MD. Pancreatoblastoma in a neonate associated with Beckwith-Wiedemann syndrome. Z Kinderchir 1986;41:56.

82. Iseki M, Suzuki T, Koizumi Y, et al. Alpha-fetoprotein–producing pancreatoblastoma. Cancer 1986;57:1833.

83. Vannier J-P, Flamant F, Hemet J, et al. Pancreatoblastoma: response to chemotherapy. Med Pediatr Oncol 1991;19:187.

84. Jaksic T, Yaman M, Thorner P, et al. A 20-year review of pediatric pancreatic tumors. J Pediatr Surg 1992;27:1315.

85. Robey G, Danceman A, Martin DJ. Pancreatic carcinoma in a neonate. Pediatr Radiol 1983;13:284.

86. Morohoshi T, Sagawa F, Mitsuya T. Pancreatoblastoma with marked elevation of serum alpha-fetoprotein. Virchows Arch [A] 1990;416:265.

87. Horie A, Yano Y, Kotoo Y, et al. Morphogenesis of pancreatoblastoma, infantile carcinoma of the pancreas. Report of two cases. Cancer 1977;39:247.

88. Silverman JF, Holbrook CT, Pories WJ, et al. Fine needle aspiration cytology of pancreatoblastoma with immunocytochemical and ultrastructural studies. Acta Cytol 1990;34:632.

89. Lack EE, Levey R, Cassady JR, et al. Tumors of the exocrine pancreas in children and adolescents. A clinical and pathologic study of eight cases. Am J Surg Pathol 1983;7:319.

90. Buchino JJ, Castello FM, Nagaraj HS. Pancreatoblastoma: a histochemical and ultrastructural analysis. Cancer 1984;53:963.

91. Frable WJ, Still WJS, Kay S. Carcinoma of the pancreas, infantile type. Cancer 1971;27:667.

92. Lopez-Kruger R, Dockerty MB. Tumors of the islets of Langerhans. Surg Gynecol Obstet 1947;85:495.

93. Creutzfeld W. Endocrine Tumors of the Pancreas. In BW Volk, FF Weldman (eds), The Diagnostic Pancreas. New York: Plenum, 1977;551.

94. Heitz PU. Pancreatic Endocrine Tumors. In G Klöppel, P Heitz (eds), Pancreatic Pathology. New York: Churchill Livingstone, 1984;206.

95. Klöppel G, Heitz PU. Pancreatic endocrine tumors. Pathol Res Pract 1988;183:155.

96. Solcia E, Capella C, Klöppel G. Tumors of the Endocrine Pancreas. In E Solcia, C Capella, G Klöppel (eds), Atlas of Tumor Pathology: Tumors of the Pancreas (3rd ed). Washington, DC: Armed Forces Institute of Pathology, 1997;145.

97. Capella C, Solcia E, Frigerio B, et al. The endocrine cells of the pancreas and related tumors. Virchows Arch [A] 1977;373:327.

98. Hammar S, Sale G. Multiple hormone producing islet cell carcinomas of the pancreas. Hum Pathol 1975;6:349.

99. Heitz PU, Kasper M, Polak JM, et al. Pancreatic endocrine tumors: immunocytochemical analysis of 125 tumors. Hum Pathol 1982;13:263.

100. Mukai K, Greider MH, Grotting JC, et al. Retrospective study of 77 pancreatic endocrine tumors using the immunoperoxidase method. Am J Surg Pathol 1982;6:387.

101. Rosai J. Pancreas and Ampullary Region. In J Rosai (ed), Ackerman's Surgical Pathology (8th ed). St. Louis: Mosby, 1996;990.

102. Capella C, Heitz PU, Höfler H, et al. Revised classification of neuroendocrine tumours of the lung, pancreas and gut. Virchows Arch 1995;425:547.

103. Graeme-Cook F, Bell DA, Flotte TJ, et al. Aneuploidy in pancreatic insulinomas does not predict malignancy. Cancer 1990;66:2365.

104. Graeme-Cook F, Nardi G, Compton CC. Immunocytochemical staining for human chorionic gonadotropin subunits does not predict malignancy in insulinomas. Am J Clin Pathol 1990;93:273.

105. Pelosi G, Zamboni G, Doglioni C, et al. Immunodetection of proliferating cell nuclear antigen assesses the growth fraction and predicts malignancy in endocrine tumors of the pancreas. Am J Surg Pathol 1992;16:1215.

106. Greider MH, DeSchryver-Kecskemeti K, Kraus FT. Psammoma bodies in endocrine tumors of the gas-

troenteropancreatic axis: a rather common occurrence. Semin Diagn Pathol 1984;1:19.

107. Guarda LA, Silva EG, Ordonez NG, et al. Clear cell islet cell tumor. Am J Clin Pathol 1983;79:512.

108. Ferreiro J, Lewin K, Herron RM, et al. Malignant islet cell tumor with rhabdomyosarcomatous differentiation. Am J Surg Pathol 1989;13:422.

109. Tomita T, Bhatia P, Gourley W. Mucin producing islet cell adenoma. Hum Pathol 1981;12:850.

110. Radi MJ, Fenoglio-Preiser CM, Chiffelle T. Functioning oncocytic islet-cell carcinoma. Am J Surg Pathol 1985;9:517.

111. Collins BT, Cramer HM. Fine-needle aspiration cytology of islet cell tumors [review]. Diagn Cytopathol 1996;15:37.

112. Al-Kaisi N, Weaver MG, Abdul KFW, et al. Fine needle aspiration cytology of neuroendocrine tumors of the pancreas. Acta Cytol 1992;36:655.

113. Sneige N, Ordonez NG, Veanattukalathil S, et al. Fine-needle aspiration cytology in pancreatic endocrine tumors. Diagn Cytopathol 1987;3:35. (Published erratum appears in Diagn Cytopathol 1987;3:176.)

114. Bell DA. Cytologic features of islet-cell tumors. Acta Cytol 1987;31:485.

115. Zalev AH, Kahn HJ, Hanna W. Fine-needle aspiration biopsy of an islet cell tumour simulating pancreatic carcinoma. Can J Surg 1988;31:429.

116. Nguyen G-K. Cytology of hyperplastic endocrine cells of the pancreas in fine needle aspiration biopsy. Acta Cytol 1984;28:499.

117. Gala I, Atkinson BF, Nicosia RF, et al. Fine-needle aspiration cytology of idiopathic pancreatic islet cell adenosis. Diagn Cytopathol 1993;9:453.

118. Banner BF, Myrent KL, Memoli VA, et al. Neuroendocrine carcinoma of the pancreas diagnosed by aspiration cytology. A case report. Acta Cytol 1985; 29:442.

119. Dodd LG, Evans DB, Symmans F, et al. Fine-needle aspiration of pancreatic extramedullary plasmacytoma: possible confusion with islet cell tumor. Diagn Cytopathol 1994;10:371.

120. Artymyshyn RL. Editorial comments: extramedullary plasmacytomas versus neuroendocrine tumors—the need for ancillary diagnostic techniques. Diagn Cytopathol 1994;10:374.

121. Cruickshank AH, Benbow EW. Pathology of the Pancreas (2nd ed). London: Springer-Verlag, 1995.

122. Corrin B, Gilby ED, Jones NF, et al. Oat cell carcinoma of the pancreas with ectopic ACTH secretion. Cancer 1973;31:1523.

123. Hobbs RD, Stewart AF, Ravin ND, et al. Hypercalcemia in small cell carcinoma of the pancreas. Cancer 1984;53:1552.

8

Metastatic Tumors of the Pancreas

Martha Bishop Pitman and Barbara A. Centeno

Secondary malignancies of the pancreas are not too uncommon, but because they seldom produce clinical symptoms, they usually go unrecognized until post-mortem examination [1, 2]. The current common practice of extensive radiologic evaluation in the metastatic workup of patients diagnosed with extrapancreatic primary malignancy has led to an increasing awareness of secondary tumors in the pancreas as well. The pancreas is a site of metastatic tumor in approximately 3–11% of patients, the most common sites of origin being the lung, breast, stomach, colon, and skin (melanoma) [1–4]. In one series, direct extension is reported as the most common cause [1], whereas another, much larger series found hematogenous spread to be most common [2]. Secondary malignancies most often present as multiple nodules but may occasionally present as solitary nodules [1, 2, 5, 6].

Fine needle aspiration biopsy (FNAB) is as useful in the evaluation of secondary pancreatic tumors as it is in primary tumors [3]. Clinicopathologic correlation, however, is essential to arriving at an accurate diagnosis.

ADENOCARCINOMA

Distinguishing a primary from a secondary adenocarcinoma is relatively impossible without clinical history. The knowledge of a preexisting tumor and comparison of the aspirated tumor with slides (cyto- or histopathology) from the patient's primary tumor are vital in making an accurate distinction. Even then, however, some cases may never be confidently resolved. With rare exceptions, there are no specific markers for adenocarcinomas to aid in the identification of the site of origin.

Breast carcinoma of the ductal type (not otherwise specified [NOS]) tends to maintain a uniform morphologic profile regardless of the site from which it is aspirated. Cells are present in flat, angulated, monolayered sheets and clusters and as single cells (Figure 8-1). Cells have a relatively low-grade appearance, with nuclear crowding, overlapping, and recognizable nuclear membrane abnormalities, but they generally lack marked anisonucleosis. Nucleoli may or may not be prominent. The cytoplasm is moderate in amount and best appreciated on single cells, where it is dense and often eccentric and cone or flame shaped (Figure 8-2). Cell-in-cell arrangements are also commonly seen in breast carcinoma (Figure 8-3). Positivity of the cells for gross cystic disease fluid protein 15 (GCDFP-15) supports an origin from the breast [7]. Estrogen receptor positivity is nonspecific because it has been detected in pancreatic carcinoma [8].

Adenocarcinomas from the *lung* metastasize far less commonly to the pancreas than do small cell carcinomas or squamous cell carcinomas [9] originating from this site. Similar to primary pancreatic adenocarcinoma, metastatic pulmonary adenocarcinoma demonstrates cellular clusters with pleomorphic nuclei, nucleoli, hyperchromasia, and cytoplasm with or without mucinous vacuolization (Figure 8-4). Both sites may demonstrate squamous differentiation, but this is more likely to be seen in lung primaries.

Metastatic adenocarcinoma of the *colon* is usually characterized by a high-grade adenocarcinoma associated with necrosis ("dirty background"), similar to its appearance in the liver [10]. The epithelial cells are columnar, with cigar-shaped, occasionally palisading, nuclei and eccentric cytoplasm (Figure 8-5).

Gastric adenocarcinoma is a diagnostic consideration in an adenocarcinoma with a prominent signet-ring cell population (Figure 8-6).

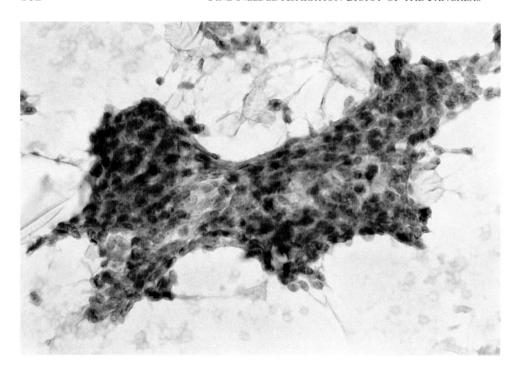

FIGURE 8-1. Metastatic breast adenocarcinoma. Flat, angulated sheet of relatively monomorphic neoplastic epithelium with peripheral dyshesion (Papanicolaou, 20×; ×1.25 optivar).

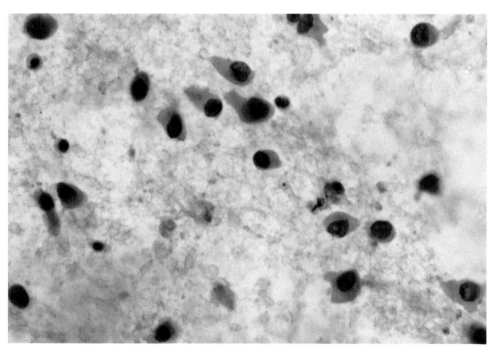

FIGURE 8-2. Metastatic breast adenocarcinoma. Numerous, relatively small and monomorphic, single malignant cells with eccentric, cone- or flame-shaped cytoplasm (Papanicolaou, 40×; ×1.6 optivar).

FIGURE 8-3. Metastatic
breast adenocarcinoma.
Malignant cells in loose
clusters, singly, and in a
cell-in-cell arrangement
(Papanicolaou, 40×; ×1.6
optivar).

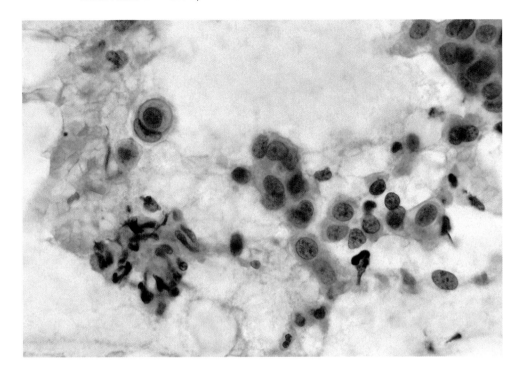

Figure 8-4. Metastatic lung
adenocarcinoma. Loose
cluster of columnar malignant cells in a pseudoglan-
dular formation. This
nonspecific morphology is
similar to pancreatic adenocarcinoma (Papanicolaou,
40×; ×1.6 optivar).

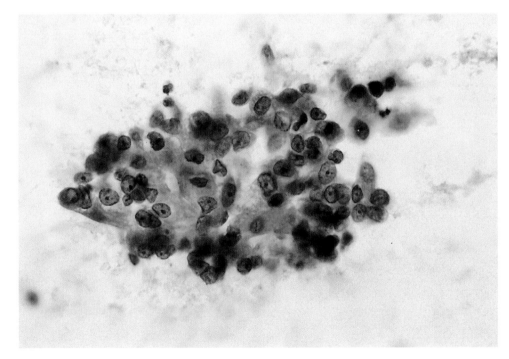

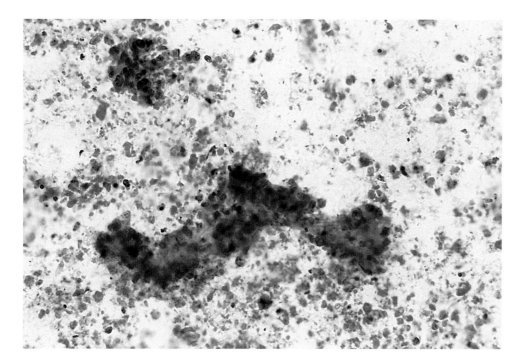

FIGURE 8-5. Metastatic colonic adenocarcinoma. Cluster of columnar cells with cigar-shaped nuclei present in a background of abundant dirty necrosis (Papanicolaou, 25×).

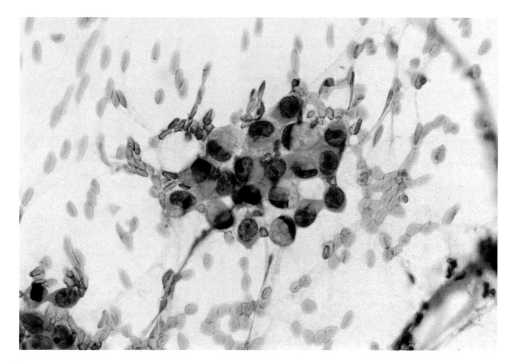

FIGURE 8-6. Metastatic signet-ring cell adenocarcinoma. Numerous signet-ring cells are suggestive of a primary gastric tumor (Papanicolaou, 40×; ×1.6 optivar).

FIGURE 8-7. Metastatic renal cell carcinoma. Loosely cohesive, flat sheet of neoplastic cells with relatively abundant, vacuolated cytoplasm and round nuclei with prominent nucleoli (Papanicolaou, 40×; ×1.6 optivar).

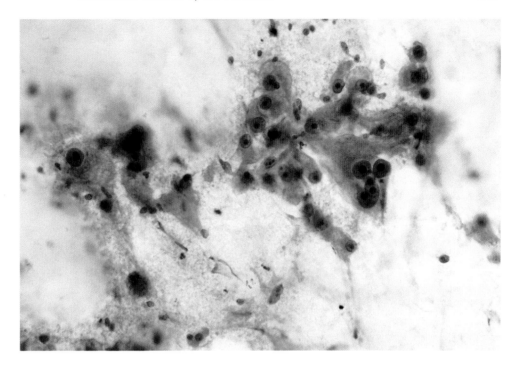

Renal cell carcinoma is the most frequently reported metastatic neoplasm to the pancreas [3, 11–21] because it is relatively unique in its ability to present many years to decades after nephrectomy. This is in contrast to most other secondary malignancies of the pancreas, which present within a year of the initial diagnosis [5]. The tumors are commonly of clear-cell type, characterized by a uniform population of polygonal clear cells with central round nuclei and prominent nucleoli (Figure 8-7).

MALIGNANT MELANOMA

Metastatic malignant melanoma is a tumor generally characterized by a predominantly dyshesive population of large cells with pleomorphic, eccentrically placed nuclei commonly adorned with macronucleoli or pseudoinclusions (Figure 8-8). The cytoplasm is ample and dense and may or may not contain melanin pigment. In the absence of melanin pigment (which is diagnostic and requires no further confirmatory studies; Figure 8-9) or other characteristic cytomorphologic features, helpful diagnostic ancillary studies include the following:

- Fontana-Masson histochemistry: Melanin granules stain black.
- Immunoperoxidase stains: Vimentin, S-100, and HMB 45 are usually positive; keratin, carcinoembryonic antigen, and other epithelial markers are negative.

- Electron microscopy: Premelanosomes, melanosomes, or both are present.

SQUAMOUS CELL CARCINOMA

The presence of a keratinizing squamous cell carcinoma on FNAB of a pancreatic mass should immediately suggest a metastasis. Although primary squamous cell carcinoma has been reported in the pancreas [22–26], the current accepted theory is that primary squamous cell carcinoma in the pancreas occurs exclusively as a component of adenosquamous carcinoma [27, 28] because thorough sectioning of primary pancreatic neoplasms presumed to be pure squamous cell carcinomas always reveal foci of glandular differentiation. Squamous cell carcinoma primaries of the lung are the most common primary site, but metastases from the esophagus [3, 4, 11], cervix [4], and tonsils [3] have also been reported. Cytomorphologic features that characterize squamous cell carcinoma include large, polygonal cells with dense (hard) cytoplasm that may or may not be keratinizing and large, pleomorphic nuclei, present both singly and in groups, and often associated with necrosis (Figure 8-10). The presence of abundant, anucleated keratotic debris has also been reported [9].

SMALL CELL CARCINOMA

The pancreas is a common site of metastasis from pulmonary small cell carcinoma [29], which needs to be dis-

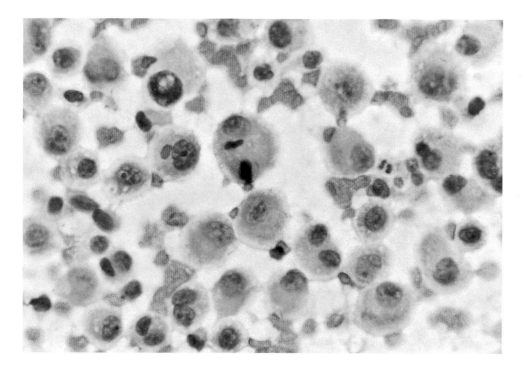

FIGURE 8-8. Metastatic malignant melanoma. Cellular smear composed of a dyshesive population of tumor cells with abundant, sharply defined cytoplasm. The nuclei are pleomorphic, with prominent nucleoli and pseudoinclusions (Papanicolaou, 40×; ×1.6 optivar).

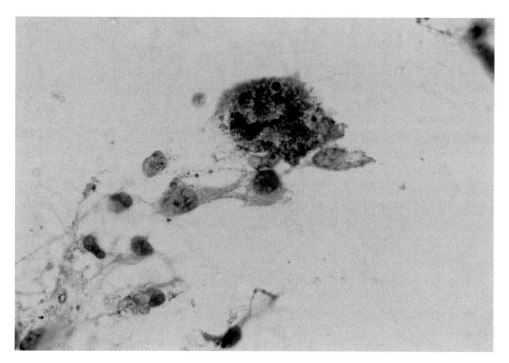

FIGURE 8-9. Metastatic malignant melanoma. Melanin pigment is visible in the cytoplasm as dusty brown pigment (Papanicolaou 40×; ×1.6 optivar).

FIGURE 8-10. Metastatic squamous cell carcinoma. Few intact, malignant keratinized cells in a background of necrotic "ghost cells" (Papanicolaou, 40×; ×1.6 optivar).

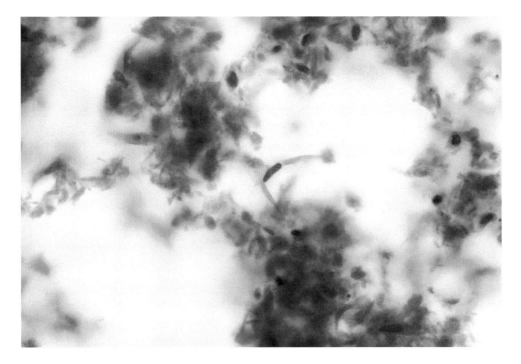

FIGURE 8-11. Metastatic small cell carcinoma. Cluster of small, hyperchromatic malignant cells with scant to invisible cytoplasm showing nuclear molding and coarse, clumped chromatin (Papanicolaou, 40×; ×1.25 optivar).

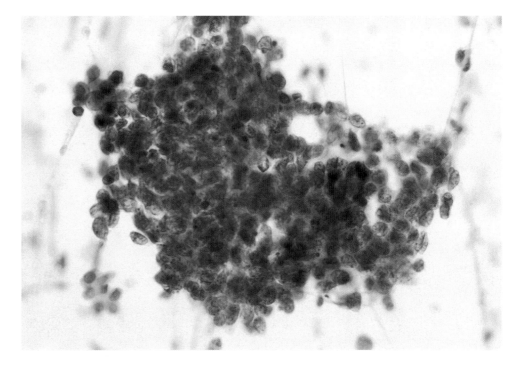

tinguished from primary pancreatic small cell carcinoma [30–32]. Given that the latter is rare, the suspicion of a metastasis should be raised when this entity is seen on pancreatic FNAB. Cytomorphologic features are typical of small cell carcinoma from any site, including small, fragile, molded cells with coarse, speckled ("neuroendocrine") chromatin and scant cytoplasm (Figure 8-11). The lack of observable cytoplasm and the presence of definite nuclear molding, nuclear pleomorphism, and

necrosis are features that help to distinguish small cell carcinoma from islet cell tumor.

MALIGNANT LYMPHOMA

Non-Hodgkin's lymphoma is the most common hematologic malignancy to involve the pancreas [2, 6]. Invariably, the involvement is secondary, with primary pancreatic lymphoma or even lymphoma predominantly

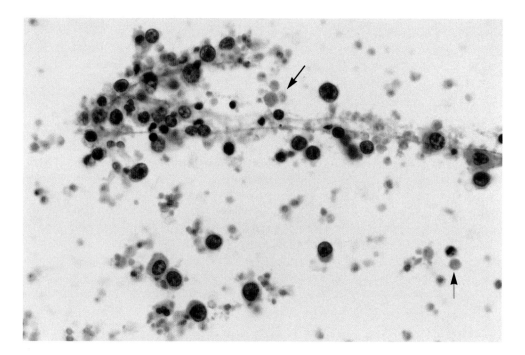

FIGURE 8-12. Malignant lymphoma, high grade. Lymphoglandular bodies (*arrow*) are small, amorphous blue globules in the background of a lymphoid population of cells, representing stripped cytoplasm (Papanicolaou, 40×; ×1.6 optivar).

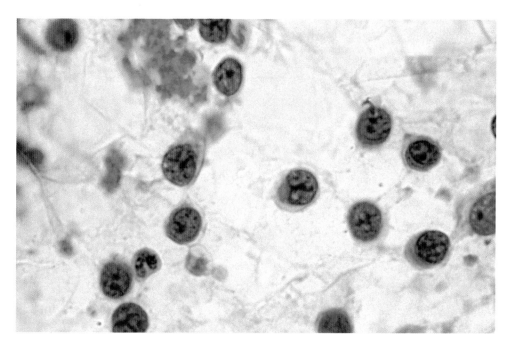

FIGURE 8-13. Malignant lymphoma, high grade. The cells have pleomorphic nuclei with irregular nuclear membranes and prominent nucleoli (Papanicolaou, 40×; ×1.6 optivar).

involving the pancreas being exceedingly rare [22, 33]. Due to the close proximity of many gastrointestinal and peripancreatic lymph nodes, direct invasion of the pancreas is common [34, 35]. The involvement of the pancreas by Hodgkin's disease, leukemia, and myeloma also occurs but is much less common [2, 4].

Aspirate smears of non-Hodgkin's lymphoma show a diffuse, single-cell population of lymphoid cells, as indicated by the presence of lymphoglandular bodies [36], a feature signifying a lymphoid rather than an epithelial tumor cell population but in no way distinguishing benign from malignant. Although lymphoglandular bodies are best visualized on air-dried Romanowsky-stained smears, they can still be appreciated on alcohol-fixed, Papanicolaou-stained slides (Figure 8-12). Large cell lymphomas are easily recognized as malignant on morphologic grounds alone due to the presence of pleomorphic nuclei with irregular nuclear membranes and, at times, prominent nucleoli (Figure 8-13).

FIGURE 8-14. Malignant lymphoma, low grade. The malignant cells are small (approximately the size of a red blood cell), relatively polymorphous, and lacking the nuclear abnormalities seen in the high-grade lymphoma shown in Figure 8-13 (Papanicolaou, 40×; ×1.25 optivar).

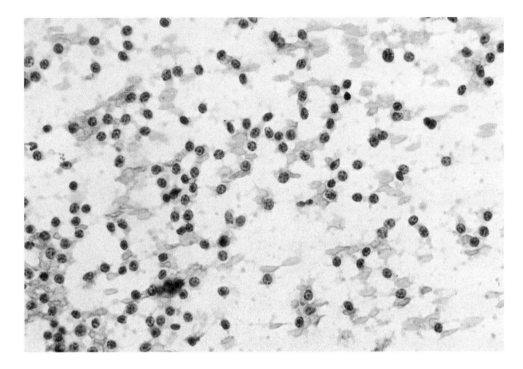

FIGURE 8-15. Metastatic mesenchymal chondrosarcoma. Uniform, loose cells with scant cytoplasm and hyperchromatic, spindle-shaped nuclei. Some of the cells have intracytoplasmic, eosinophilic material that displaces the nuclei (Hematoxylin and Eosin, 40×; ×1.6 optivar).

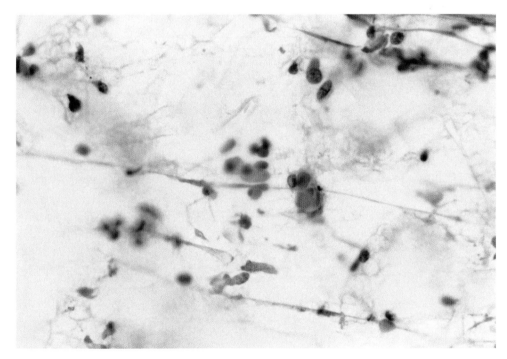

Low-grade lymphomas, such as follicular center cell or marginal zone lymphomas (Figure 8-14), may require marker studies to determine clonality. This can be done either by immunocytochemistry performed on smears or cell block preparations or by flow cytometry. The FNAB diagnosis of lymphoma is one of the most important diagnoses to make because it prompts immediate treatment and spares the patient unnecessary surgery.

RARE AND UNUSUAL METASTASES

It is conceivable that just about any tumor can metastasize to the pancreas. Case reports of rare metastases to the pancreas include phyllodes tumor [3], dedifferentiated chondrosarcoma [37], leiomyosarcoma [38], choriocarcinoma [2], and medulloblastoma [39]. We have seen examples of metastatic mesenchymal chondrosarcoma (Figure 8-15),

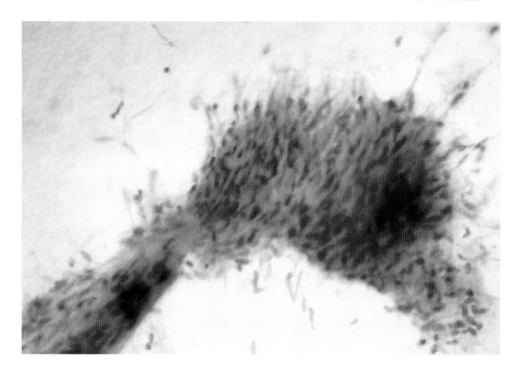

Figure 8-16. Leiomyosarcoma. Smears contain cellular sheets of malignant overlapping, spindled cells with blunt-ended nuclei (Papanicolaou, 10×).

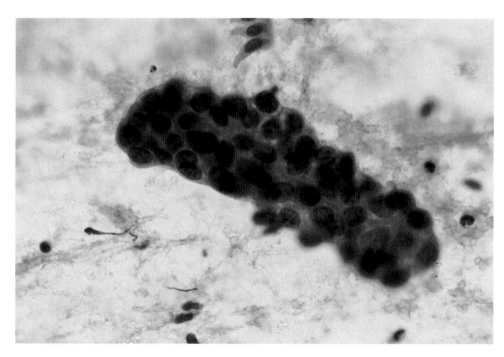

Figure 8-17. Metastatic ovarian papillary serous cystadenocarcinoma, represented by a three-dimensional papillary cluster of malignant cells (Papanicolaou, 40×; ×1.6 optivar).

leiomyosarcoma (Figure 8-16), and papillary serous carcinoma of the ovary (Figure 8-17).

REFERENCES

1. Willis RA. The Spread of Tumours in the Human Body (3rd ed). London: Butterworth, 1973.

2. Cubilla AL, Fitzgerald PJ. Cancer (Nonendocrine) of the Pancreas: A Suggested Classification. In PJ Fitzgerald, AB Morrison (eds), The Pancreas. Baltimore: Williams & Wilkins, 1980.

3. Carson HJ, Green LK, Castelli MJ, et al. Utilization of fine-needle aspiration biopsy in the diagnosis of metastatic tumors to the pancreas. Diagn Cytopathol 1995;12:8.

4. Benning TL, Silverman JF, Berns LA, et al. Fine needle aspiration of metastatic and hematologic malignancies clinically mimicking pancreatic carcinoma. Acta Cytol 1992;36:471.

5. Robbins EG II, Franceschi D, Barkin JS. Solitary metastatic tumors to the pancreas: a case report and review of the literature [review]. Am J Gastroenterol 1996;91:2414.

6. Cruickshank AH, Benbow EW. Secondary Tumours, Lymphomas and Rare Tumours. In AH Cruickshank, EW Benbow (eds), Pathology of the Pancreas (2nd ed). New York: Springer-Verlag, 1995;219.

7. Kaufmann O, Deidesheimer T, Muehlenberg M, et al. Immunohistochemical differentiation of metastatic breast carcinomas from metastatic adenocarcinoma of other primary sites. Histopathology 1996;29:233.

8. Andren-Sandberg A, Borg S, Dawiskiba I, et al. Estrogen receptors and estrogen binding protein in pancreatic cancer. Digestion 1982;25:12.

9. Mockli GC, Silversmith M. Squamous cell carcinoma of the lung metastatic to the pancreas: diagnosis by fine-needle aspiration biopsy. Diagn Cytopathol 1997;16:287.

10. Pitman MB, Szyfelbein WM. Fine Needle Aspiration Biopsy of the Liver. Boston: Butterworth–Heinemann, 1994.

11. Biset JM, Laurent F, de Verbizier G, et al. Ultrasound and computed tomographic findings in pancreatic metastases. Eur J Radiol 1991;12:41.

12. Temellini F, Bavosi M, Lamarra M, et al. Pancreatic metastasis 25 years after nephrectomy for renal cancer. Tumori 1989;75:503.

13. Fullarton GM, Burgoyne M. Gallbladder and pancreatic metastases from bilateral renal carcinoma presenting with hematobilia and anemia. Urology 1991;38:184.

14. Rypens F, Van Gansbeke D, Lambilliotte JP, et al. Pancreatic metastasis from renal cell carcinoma. Br J Radiol 1992;65:547.

15. Jenssen E. A metastatic hypernephroma to the pancreas. Eur J Surg Suppl 1952;104:177.

16. Franciosi RA, Russo JF. Renal cell carcinoma metastasis to the pancreas thirteen years following nephrectomy. Mil Med 1969;134:200.

17. Guttman FM, Ross M, Lachance C. Pancreatic metastasis of renal cell carcinoma treated by total pancreatectomy. Arch Surg 1972;105:782.

18. Saxon A, Gottesman J, Doolas A. Bilateral hypernephroma with solitary pancreatic metastasis. J Surg Oncol 1980;13:317.

19. Yazaki T, Ishikawa S, Ogawa Y, et al. Silent pancreatic metastasis from renal cell carcinoma diagnosed at arteriography. Acta Urol Jpn 1981;27:1517.

20. Weerdenburg JP, Jurgens PJ. Late metastasis of a hypernephroma to the thyroid and the pancreas. Diagn Imaging Clin Med 1984;53:269.

21. Gohji K, Matsumoto O, Kamidono S. Solitary pancreatic metastasis from renal cell carcinoma. Hinyokika Kiyo 1990;36:677.

22. Cubilla AL, Fitzgerald PJ. Tumors of the Exocrine Pancreas. Atlas of Tumor Pathology, Fascicle

19. Washington, DC: Armed Forces Institute of Pathology, 1984;136, 168.

23. Brayko CM, Doll DC. Squamous cell carcinoma of the pancreas associated with hypercalcemia. Gastroenterology 1982;83:1297.

24. Fajardo LL, Yoshino MT, Chernin MM. Computed tomography findings in squamous cell carcinoma of the pancreas. J Comput Assist Tomogr 1982;12:138.

25. Morgan J, Amazon K, Termin L. Squamous cell carcinoma infiltrating a pancreatic pseudocyst. South Med J 1989;82:1161.

26. Sears HF, Kim Y, Strawitz J. Squamous cell carcinoma of the pancreas. J Surg Oncol 1980;14:261.

27. Klöppel G, Solcia E, Longnecker DS, et al. Histological Typing of Tumours of the Exocrine Pancreas (2nd ed). Berlin: Springer-Verlag, 1996.

28. Cihak RW, Kawashima T, Steer A. Adenoacanthoma (adenosquamous carcinoma) of the pancreas. Cancer 1972;29:1133.

29. Matthews MJ. Problems in Morphology and Behavior of Bronchopulmonary Malignant Disease. In L Israel, AP Chahinian (eds), Lung Cancer: Natural History, Prognosis, and Therapy. New York: Academic, 1976;52.

30. Banner BF, Myrent KL, Memoli VA, et al. Neuroendocrine carcinoma of the pancreas diagnosed by aspiration cytology. A case report. Acta Cytol 1985;29:442.

31. Reyes CV, Wang T. Undifferentiated small cell carcinoma of the pancreas: a report of five cases. Cancer 1981;47:2500.

32. Bommer KK, Laucirica R, Schwartz MR. Fine needle aspiration cytology of pancreatic small cell carcinoma. Acta Cytol 1994;38:857.

33. Cappell MS, Yao F, Cho KC, et al. Lymphoma predominantly involving the pancreas. Dig Dis Sci 1989;34:942.

34. Ehrlich AN, Stadler G, Geller W, et al. Gastrointestinal manifestations of malignant lymphoma. Gastroenterology 1968;54:1115.

35. Wright DH. Gross Distribution and Haematology. In DP Burkitt, DH Wright (eds), Burkitt's Lymphoma. Edinburgh: Livingstone, 1970;248.

36. Soderstrom N. The free cytoplasmic fragments of lymphoglandular tissue (lymphoglandular bodies). Scand J Haematol 1968;5:138.

37. Mikhail MGS, Lim KB. Dedifferentiated chondrosarcoma metastasizing to the pancreas in pregnancy. Acta Obstet Gynecol Scand 1989;68:467.

38. Holmes GF, Ali SZ. Fine-needle aspiration of leiomyosarcoma metastatic to the pancreas. Diagn Cytopathol 1997;16:189.

39. Krouwer HG, Vollmer Havsen J, White J, et al. Desmoplastic medulloblastoma metastatic to the pancreas: case report. Neurosurgery 1991;29:612.

9

Specimen Preparation Techniques

David P. Beech

At Massachusetts General Hospital, a rapid interpretation of all radiologically guided biopsies is performed. The role of cytotechnologists is exciting and challenging, as they are the first to arrive on the scene, where they must rapidly prepare the slides and evaluate specimen adequacy. The cytotechnologist calls the cytopathologist at the appropriate time, who then issues a statement of adequacy, a preliminary diagnosis and, if necessary, requests tissue for special studies, such as a lymphoma workup.

CLINICAL INFORMATION

In our laboratory, a great emphasis is placed on obtaining the patient's clinical diagnosis and history. Before evaluating the aspiration, we obtain past diagnoses via previous cytology and pathology reports, treatment history, and any available relevant glass slides for comparison. Important current clinical and radiologic information includes the size of the lesion, its location, whether it is a solitary nodule or one of multiple nodules, whether the clinical suspicion is of a primary lesion or a metastasis, radiologic findings, whether the lesion is solid or cystic, and if the latter, whether it is unilocular or multilocular or associated with a solid area. The gathering of this history is vital for an accurate, rapid interpretation and for subsequent diagnosis on the final slides.

PREPARATION OF RAPID SMEARS

The cytotechnologist travels to the designated area in the radiology department when alerted. A mobile aspiration biopsy kit is carried to the reading room, where a temporary laboratory is set up. Microscopes are conveniently stored there for this purpose. The contents of the aspira-

tion biopsy kit include water baths, stains, xylene, mounting media, coverslips, paper clips (which keep slides separate in the jar of alcohol fixative), gauze pads (to drain excess xylene and mounting media), and dotting pens.

After each aspiration, the radiologist expresses a small amount of the specimen (about two drops) on a frosted glass slide. The specimen is smeared using the pull-apart method [1] because it is the method our cytotechnologists are most familiar and comfortable with, but any smear technique that provides well-preserved, noncrushed material can be used. A clean frosted slide is placed over the one containing the specimen, and the material is gently pressed together so as not to crush the sample or strip nuclei of their cytoplasm. The cellular material is pulled away from the labeled end. The two slides are pulled apart and immediately immersed into a fixative of 5% glacial acetic acid and 95% ethyl alcohol, which achieves rapid fixation and lysis of excess blood. Paper clips are used to keep the slides separated in the jar of fixative. The slides are fixed for a minimum of 30 seconds, and one slide from each pair is stained using the rapid Hematoxylin and Eosin (H&E) staining technique [2] (Table 9-1).

THE RAPID INTERPRETATION

The cytotechnologist screens the slide or slides for adequacy, appropriateness of anatomic site, and the presence of malignancy. If the slide has only benign material, the radiologist may choose to re-aspirate. Once the slides are considered diagnostic of a lesion (benign or malignant), the cytotechnologist calls for the cytopathologist, who again determines adequacy and renders a rapid interpretation.

Table 9-1. Rapid Hematoxylin and Eosin Stain

Procedure	Duration
1. Fix in solution of 5% glacial acetic acid in 95% ethyl alcohol.	30 secs
2. Wash in distilled water.	2 dips
3. Rinse in acid-water solution.[a]	2 dips
4. Stain in hematoxylin.[b]	30 secs
5. Rinse in distilled water.	3 dips
6. Differentiate in acid-water solution.	2 dips
7. "Blue" immediately in tap water to raise the pH of the stained material and change the color from red-purple to blue.	4–5 dips
8. Wash in distilled water.	10 dips
9. Counterstain in alcoholic Eosin.[c]	3–5 dips
10. Dehydrate in 95% ethyl alcohol.	5 dips
11. Dehydrate in 99% isopropyl alcohol.	5 dips
12. Clear in xylene.	5–10 dips
13. Mount the slide with mounting medium and coverslip.	—

[a]Acid-water solution of 2 ml glacial acetic acid in 250 ml distilled water.
[b]Hematoxylin: Gill 3 (triple strength) Hematoxylin (Lerner Laboratories, Fisher Scientific, Orangeburg, NY). Be sure to add 2–3 ml glacial acetic acid to each 250 ml of fresh dye solution.
[c]Eosin Y, 1% alcohol solution (Harelco Brand, EM Diagnostic Systems, Gibbstown, NJ). Dilute with equal volume of 95% ethyl alcohol. Add 2 ml glacial acetic acid to each 250 ml of staining solution.

PREPARATION OF SLIDES FOR FINAL INTERPRETATION

The remainder of slides not stained by rapid H&E are labeled with the patient's name and placed into 95% ethyl alcohol until they are ready to be stained by the Papanicolaou (Pap) method [3] (Table 9-2). Air-dried smears are not routinely prepared on pancreatic aspirates because the vast majority of pancreatic lesions are epithelial and require nuclear detail for proper evaluation. Air-dried smears are prepared only if requested at the time of rapid interpretation. Needle rinsings suspended in saline are collected and processed with a cytospin or ThinPrep processor (Cytyc Corporation, Boxborough, MA), or both. For cytospins, the sample is transferred to 50-ml centrifuge tubes and centrifuged at 600 gravities (1,500 rpm) for 10 minutes. The supernatant is poured off, and the cell pellet is resuspended by vortex in 5 ml of Hank's balanced salt solution. Cytospin chambers are assembled, and 5–7 drops of the resuspended sample are placed within the chambers, centrifuged for 1 minute at 1,250 rpm, and fixed in 95% ethanol. For ThinPrep slides, the sample is transferred to a 50-ml centrifuge tube, and 30 ml of Cytolyt solution is added. The sample is centrifuged at 600 gravities for 10 minutes. The supernatant is poured off, and the pellet is resuspended by vortex. If there is no visible pellet, an aliquot of PreservCyt Solution is poured from the vial into the tube, the tube vortexed to mix, and the sample poured back into the vial. If sediment is visible. two drops of the sample are pipetted into a 20-ml PreservCyt Solution vial. The specimen is incubated for 5 minutes. The slide is then made with the ThinPrep Processor. The specimen is fixed in 95% ethyl alcohol until it is ready to be stained by the Pap method.

Tissue core fragments that have been obtained are removed and placed into a centrifuge tube containing 10% formalin and sent for routine histologic processing. The needle rinsings can be used for additional cytospin or ThinPrep slides if an adequate core is available for cell block. These extra slides may be used for special studies if a cell button is inadequate for cell block or core samples proved inadequate for diagnosis or special studies.

TABLE 9-2. Routine Papanicolaou Stain

Station Number	Solution	Time (min)
1	Running water	1.0
2	Hematoxylin[a]	2.0
3	Running water	1.0
4	Running water	1.0
5	96% ethanol	2.0
6	Orange G[b]	1.0
7	95% ethanol	2.0
8	Eosin polychrome[c] (EA)	6.0
9	95% ethanol[d]	4.0
10	95% ethanol	3.0
11	95% ethanol	2.0
12	99% isopropanol	3.0
13	Xylene	2.0
14	Xylene	2.0

[a]Gill Hematoxylin stain. Mix all of the following ingredients on magnetic stirrer for 1 hour. All ingredients must be dissolved. Stain may be used immediately.

Distilled water	710 ml
Ethyl glycol	250 ml
Hematoxylin (color index #75290)	2.0 g
Sodium iodate ($NaIO_3$)	0.2 g (Accurate weight is critical.)
Aluminum sulfate ($Al_2SO_4 \cdot 18\ H_2O$)	17.0 g
Glacial acetic acid	40.0 ml

[b]Orange G stain: Gill formula.

1. Stock solution (0.2 M). Dissolve 9.05 g actual dye in 100 ml distilled water. 9.05 g ÷ percentage of dye content = weight.
2. Orange G working solution. Mix all of the following ingredients. Stain may be used immediately.

0.2 M stock Orange G	10 ml
Phosphotungstic acid	1 g
95% ethyl alcohol	985 ml
Glacial acetic acid	5 ml

[c]Eosin polychrome: Gill formula.

1. Stock solutions. Dissolve the following in 100 ml distilled water (70–80°C):

0.4 M light green SF yellowish (color index #42095)	3.17 g actual dye
0.30 M Eosin Y (color index #45380)	20.8 g actual dye
0.04 M fast green FCF (color index #42053)	3.24 g actual dye

2. Working solution for slides. Mix together the following:

0.04 M light green SF yellowish	10 ml
0.30 M Eosin Y	20 ml
Phosphotungstic acid	2.0 g
95% ethyl alcohol	700 ml
Absolute methyl alcohol	250 ml
Glacial acetic acid	20 ml

[d]Change 95% ethanol of Station 9 between staining runs.

THE LYMPHOMA WORKUP

If lymphoma is suspected, needle rinsings are obtained for flow cytometry, and core biopsy specimens are obtained if possible. Flow cytometry is the method of choice for immunophenotyping because it is quick and reliable when an adequate sample is obtained. The core biopsies are also used for immunophenotyping, and they may provide additional information about architecture.

In the flow cytometry laboratory, the needle rinsings are prepared according to standard techniques [4]. The panel routinely used to assess monoclonality includes T-cell antigens (CD3, CD4, CD8), B-cell antigens (CD 5, 10, 19, 20, and 23), and kappa and lambda light chains. Keratins may be added if the differential diagnosis includes carcinoma. Tissue cores are placed in saline and taken to the frozen section laboratory, where the specimen is either entirely frozen or divided between frozen tissue, B-5–fixed tissue, and formalin. If only a small amount of tissue is available, it is all frozen. An initial frozen section is cut to determine adequacy for immunohistochemical studies. If the cores are adequate, several frozen sections are cut and placed on albumin-covered, clear glass slides for immunohistochemical studies. The panel includes a standard Pan B-cell and T-cell marker and kappa and lambda. Other antibodies are added as needed for further subtyping. If cores are not available for immunohistochemical studies or flow cytometry studies were not done on the needle rinsings, the needle rinsings may be spun down into cytospin slides for immunocytochemical evaluation of cell surface antigens. One cytospin is air dried and stained with Diff Quik (Baxter Healthcare Products, Miami) (Table 9-3), and four to six cytospin slides are prepared, air-dried, dipped briefly in acetone, air-dried again, and frozen for immunoperoxidase studies. Monoclonality cannot be assessed on destained smear preparations.

PREPARATION OF PANCREATIC CYSTS

When pancreatic cysts are received in the laboratory, the undiluted sample is centrifuged if its volume is more than 1.0 ml. If it is less than that, the sample is diluted with Hank's balanced salt solution, and the volume of the diluting liquid and the original volume received are recorded so that the chemistry laboratory can make use of correction factors for its analyses. The supernatant is stored frozen and sent to the chemistry laboratory for analysis of tumor markers, including carcinoembryonic antigen, CA 125, CA 15.3, CA 72-4, tissue polypeptide antigen, pancreatic enzymes and isoenzymes, and viscosity (these are discussed in greater detail in Chapter 6). Depending on the cellularity of the centrifuged specimen pellet, the following preparations are made:

1. Four alcohol-fixed cytocentrifuge slides are prepared. These can be used for Pap stain and cytochemical stains (typically mucicarmine and alcian blue).
2. One ThinPrep slide is prepared. *Caution:* ThinPrep processing may dissolve the mucin present. Cytospins should be used for Pap and cytochemical stains if no neoplastic cells are present on ThinPrep slide.
3. One cell block. If there is enough sample to make a cell block, it may also be used to make slides for extra studies.

OTHER SPECIAL STUDIES

Estrogen-Progesterone Receptors

If the lesion is clinically or morphologically suspicious for metastatic breast cancer, direct smears can be processed for markers of the estrogen-progesterone receptors (Abbott ER-ICA Monoclonal, Abbott Laboratories, Abbott Park, IL) (Table 9-4).

Electron Microscopy

If the tumor is a poorly differentiated carcinoma, a sarcoma, or other undifferentiated tumor, either a core biopsy specimen or an aspirate specimen can be fixed in glutaraldehyde for electron microscopy. For the latter, needle rinsings are centrifuged and the pellet fixed in glu-

TABLE 9-3. Diff Quik Stain on Air-Dried Material (Plain Glass Slides Only)

1. Methanol	5 dips
2. Solution I	5 dips
3. Solution II	5 dips
4. Distilled water	5–6 dips
5. Dry slides, mount with coverslip	—

TABLE 9-4. Estrogen or Progesterone Receptor Protocol

1. 4% formaldehyde	10–15 mins
2. Phosphate-buffered saline (PBS)	5 mins
3. Cold methanol	4 mins
4. Cold acetone	3 mins
5. PBS	5 mins
6. Storage buffer	Until stained

TABLE 9-5. Special Studies

Stain	Fixative	Slide Type	Use of Destained Papanicolaou Smear
Papanicolaou	95% ethanol Acid alcohol	Plain or frosted	—
Fontana-Masson	95% ethanol Acid alcohol Formalin	Plain or frosted	Yes
Mucicarmine	95% ethanol Acid alcohol Formalin	Plain or frosted	Yes
Alcian blue	95% ethanol Acid alcohol Formalin	Plain or frosted	Yes
Periodic acid–Schiff	95% ethanol Acid alcohol Formalin	Plain or frosted	Yes
Grocott-methenamine silver	95% ethanol Acid alcohol Formalin	Plain or frosted	Yes
Chromogranin	95% ethanol Acid alcohol Formalin	Plain or frosted	Yes
Diff-Quik	Air dry	Plain	No
Lymphoid series immunocytochemistry (kappa, lambda CD3, IgG, IgM, CD22)	Air dry	Plain	No
Immunocytochemistry for nonlymphoid neoplasms (carcinoembryonic antigen, alpha-fetoprotein, alpha$_1$-antitrypsin, cytokeratins)	95% ethanol Acid alcohol Formalin	Plain or frosted	—
S-100	Formalin Air dry	Plain	No

taraldehyde. Electron microscopy is particularly helpful for patients who have no known primary malignancy.

DESTAINING

Slides stained by the Pap method or rapid H&E must be destained for some special stains and immunocytochemistry (Table 9-5). Our destaining method is as follows:

1. The coverslip is removed by placing the slide in xylene until the coverslip falls off.
2. The slide is rinsed in two changes of xylene for 3 minutes each.
3. The slide is rinsed in 99% isopropyl alcohol or absolute ethyl alcohol for 3 minutes.
4. The slide is rinsed in 95% ethyl alcohol and concentrated hydrochloric acid (2 ml hydrochloric acid to 100 ml ethyl alcohol) for

10–15 minutes with occasional dipping (check for decolorization, and repeat if necessary).
5. The slide is placed in 95% ethyl alcohol until it is restained with the desired special stain.

REFERENCES

1. Takahashi M. Color Atlas of Cancer Cytology (2nd ed). Tokyo: Igako-Shoin, 1981;74.
2. Pierce A. A Manual for Histologic Technicians (3rd ed). Boston: Little, Brown, 1972;100.
3. Gill GW, Miller KA. Laboratory Cytopathology Techniques for Specimen Preparation. Baltimore: Johns Hopkins Hospital, Cytopathology Department, 1973.
4. Preffer FI. Flow Cytometry. In RB Colvin, AK Bahn, RT McCluskey (eds), Diagnostic Immunopathology. New York: Raven, 1995;733.

Index